THE HEART OF REIKI

BY DR. SUSAN DOWNING, PH.D.

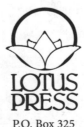

LOTUS
PRESS

P.O. Box 325
Twin Lakes, WI 53181 USA

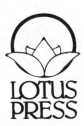

LOTUS
PRESS

Lotus Press

P.O. Box 325

Twin Lakes, WI 53181 USA

800-824-6396 (toll free order phone)

262-889-8561 (office phone)

262-889-2461 (office fax)

www.lotuspress.com (website)

lotuspress@lotuspress.com (email)

TABLE OF CONTENTS

EXPRESSION OF GRATITUDE

It is only thanks to a great many people and fortunate circumstances in my life that I was able to conceive of and write this book. My first bow of thanks goes to Reiki's founder Mikao Usui, without whom I would never have encountered Reiki. I also want to thank all my students, especially Fred Olson, for your sincere engagement with Reiki and for all that you have taught *me*. Thank you to Jeffrey Brooks and Karen Olander for being so generous with your time and for offering such insightful suggestions on the manuscript, and to Pamela Downing for consultation on the Japanese meaning of the precepts. My readers — and I — are fortunate, indeed, that you all agreed to help.

To my parents, Ruth and Paul Downing: thank you for teaching me how important it is to be compassionate and take care of others, for passing along the genes have helped me steadfastly pursue this life's work, and for always supporting me as I've done so. Thank you to my extended family — Mike, Emily and Peter Scotto, Pamela Downing, and Maia and Zoe Stack — for sharing my enthusiasm for Reiki and for giving me the honor of teaching some of you to practice it, too. Bev Matakaetis: thank goodness you encouraged me to learn Reiki and gave me the gift of a purposeful way to use it, right from the start. Special thanks to Karen Olander, my dear friend and Reiki Master Teacher. How fortunate I have been to have you teach me with such skill, love and care. Your friendship and support mean the world to me, and your insight into Reiki, and all of our discussions have been instrumental in helping my Reiki practice grow and mature. Finally, I offer deepest thanks to my teacher and friend, Jeffrey Brooks. You have guided my study and practice of the Dharma and shown me, by example, how to bring my bodhisattva vows to bear in my life. By helping my Buddhist practice blossom and deepen, you made it possible for me to grasp the connection between my Reiki and Buddhist practices. Without your friendship, encouragement and guidance, this book would never have been written. I dedicate it to you.

I bow to you all in deepest gratitude.

INTRODUCTION

The secret of inviting happiness through many blessings
The spiritual medicine for all illness

Just for today:
Do not be angry
Do not worry
Express gratitude
Devote yourself diligently to your work
Be kind to people

Do Gassho every morning and evening
Repeat the precepts and keep them in your mind and heart
To improve your body and mind

— Mikao Usui

"The secret method of inviting happiness." That's how Mikao Usui, who developed and taught Reiki in Japan in the 1920s, described the method we call Reiki. But what, exactly, did he mean by "happiness"?

Although we don't know all the specifics of how Usui Sensei worked with his students, we do know that his overarching purpose was to help them — and, by extension, us — experience personal or spiritual transformation. I've come to see Usui Sensei's words as a concise expression of his purpose. He seems to be saying, "If you practice as I have taught, you will experience transformation, and as a result of that transformation, great happiness will arise."

The five precepts Usui Sensei gives us here are certainly part of the method he taught for achieving happiness. If we do not give in to anger, if we do not worry, if we strive to be grateful and diligent and kind, then certainly we will see our lives change for the better over time: we will improve our body and mind. But that's not all. We can also see the precepts as an expression of what we'll be capable of once we've invited that happiness in: we'll feel less anger and worry, which will enable us to feel more gratitude, devote ourselves more diligently to our calling, and be kinder to others. But still, the question remains: what precisely is this happiness that we can invite into our lives by practicing Reiki, and that can bring us all these other benefits?

An answer to this question came to me only after I had devoted myself to living a life of integrated Reiki and Buddhist practice. Over a period of years, I consciously and unconsciously drew elements of my Buddhist practice into my Reiki work, until finally the two marvelously and unexpectedly came together: I found that as I gave Reiki to others, great compassion would arise in me, followed by deep happiness. This joy would spread outward in all directions, benefiting not only me, but those around me, too. I am sure that it was *this* happiness Usui Sensei had in mind.

This happiness arises in response to the great compassion that develops and deepens as the heart and mind undergo transformation. Call it personal transformation or spiritual transformation, but what lies at its heart is *our heart*: the more love and compassion we feel in our heart, the greater our happiness will be, and the easier it will be for us to share that love and happiness with those around us. I believe that the way Usui Sensei taught his students to practice enabled them to transform their minds so that great compassion would naturally grow in their hearts, and reside there to both call forth and sustain an ever-deepening happiness.

Having understood what Usui Sensei was striving to help his students experience, and having discovered through my own practice that this is possible, I want to share the fruits of my own work with you. What I've heard students and colleagues say about practicing Reiki — that the happiness they feel after giving or receiving Reiki is temporary, fading within hours or days — has led me to believe others could benefit from the practice I've developed. That's why I wrote *The Heart of Reiki*: so that you, too, can learn to practice Reiki in a way that will transform your heart and mind and invite this deep, strong and enduring happiness into your life.

The Heart of Reiki presents the framework I created based on my own experience. I do not claim that this is the way Usui Sensei worked with his students. I can't know whether or not that's the case, but I can say that Usui Sensei's example has always inspired my own practice, and I believe that what I offer you here is in the spirit of his purpose and teachings. And although this framework grew out of my own work with Reiki and Buddhist teachings, it is suitable for practitioners of any spiritual orientation, and with any level of Reiki training.

The point of this practice is to help you experience personal transformation, not to give you techniques to enhance a professional Reiki practice, or hints about how to work more effectively on others. Although the Heart of Reiki framework does include sharing Reiki with a practice partner, this practice is for *you*, for *your* development. As you move through this practice, you'll be giving Reiki to yourself and a practice partner or volunteer; learning energy practice/meditations; and reflecting on Usui Sensei's precepts.

In this practice you don't consciously figure anything out or decide what emotions or issues to address. Rather, by placing your focus on engaging in the practice consistently and sincerely, little by little, you will begin to experience benefits and transformation. Your compassion will grow, and the disturbing emotions that are preventing you from experiencing the happiness that is patiently waiting to flow into your life will gradually fade. As well, you'll see that you can not only transform your daily life with this practice, but also draw on it for support as you move through life's difficult moments.

This book will guide you at every step along this path. In Chapter One ("A Path to Happiness") I'll tell you how I came to understand Usui Sensei's teachings, as I pursued my own Reiki and Buddhist practices. That will give you an idea of the essence of the Heart of Reiki practice. Chapter Two ("Is This Path for You?") will help you decide whether this practice might be a good fit for you. Chapter Three ("Preparing for Your Journey") explains what practice elements you'll be learning, and gives suggestions for how to find a practice partner and set up a workable practice routine and schedule. The actual practice instructions begin in Chapter Four ("Stage One Practice",) which lays out the first of the six Heart of Reiki practice stages. As you continue to make your way through these stages, in Chapters Seven to Eleven, you'll also learn how to evaluate your progress (Chapter Five: "Gauging Your Progress") and how to use your practice when life's challenges throw you off balance (Chapter Six: "Using Your Practice to Survive Turmoil".) Finally, Chapter Twelve ("The Heart of Reiki In Your Professional Practice") explains how to incorporate the Heart of Reiki elements into your Reiki sessions, once you've laid that stable foundation of happiness in your own life.

You can embark on this transformative journey no matter what level of Reiki training you've had, and no matter what spiritual beliefs you do or don't hold. All you need is the desire to invite great happiness into your life. And so, I invite you to read further and join me on this joyous path!

CHAPTER ONE

A Path to Happiness

When I began practicing Reiki, I wasn't thinking about what Usui Sensei had meant by happiness. I'd decided to learn Reiki as part of my hospice volunteer training: our instructor told us how comforting Reiki was to hospice patients and offered us Level I training. Since I had also been accepted to nursing school and would start those classes in a few months, I figured Reiki would be a useful addition to my box of healing tools.

When I said yes to that first level, I knew almost nothing about Reiki. I'd heard the word, but I'd never had a session. Even so, almost as soon as class began, I was strongly drawn to Reiki. It felt as though I was remembering Reiki, not learning it. And I was happy to learn that Usui Sensei had been a Buddhist, because I myself practice Buddhism and at that time was studying intensely, in the midst of preparing to take bodhisattva vows.

Within Buddhism, bodhisattvas are beings who, out of great love and compassion, devote themselves to ending the suffering of sentient beings and to developing the wisdom and skill that will enable them to do this. "Bodhicitta" is the Sanskrit word for this special compassion itself, but is also refers to the intention this love brings forth in you to reach enlightenment so you can help others end their suffering, too. People who are inspired to emulate bodhisattvas, as I am, can take bodhisattva vows, through which you dedicate this and all future lives to working to relieve the suffering of all beings. When I received Reiki training, I couldn't have explained why Reiki seemed like a perfect fit with my Buddhist practice and my plans to take these vows. I just *felt* it. I sensed that practicing Reiki was the key to something for me.

I was able to begin using Reiki right away, and frequently, with dying patients. Both the joy that giving Reiki brought to me and the comfort the patients received amazed me. Although I wasn't thinking at all about how Usui Sensei had described his method, I was already experiencing the happiness that comes from being able to share a loving connection with others through Reiki. Little did I know that the delight I gained in my first experiences with Reiki would only grow and become more profound and transformative as I committed myself more and more to Reiki, as I ceased thinking of Reiki as just one more tool and instead saw it grow into my life's practice.

That shift in focus began on the level of non-conscious thought. One night, not long after my Reiki I training, I had a dream. I'd never been one to pay attention to dreams or to use them to guide my life decisions, but this one really intrigued me. In the dream, I walked into a classroom in an old building, which although it was set up with traditional wooden student desks, also seemed to double as both an art supply store and a doctor's waiting room. For some reason, I began to pass the time by working on a Christmas stocking. It was all sewn together, but I wanted to find just the right implement to write a name on the stocking's white cuff. I tried various magic markers, but none seemed like the right tool.

Still looking, I walked over to a tall oak counter, one like you'd see in old stores. I spotted bunches of colored pencils, but all of them had clearly been used, since they were of varying lengths and somewhat worn down. None of them seemed like suitable tools, either.

Then a man behind the counter, seeing that I was looking for something, said, "Here, take a look at this." He slid open a clear plastic bin, pulled out a handful of rocks of various sizes, and placed them on the counter in front of me. They were the color of dirt, but with yellow golden patches and some rich brown patches as well. The man took one in his two hands and manipulated it somehow, and suddenly a baby alligator emerged from it. He repeated the process with two different rocks and produced two tiny baby elephants. They smiled — can elephants smile? — and walked over to me. I petted them, then put my face down to nuzzle them.

Next, the man came out from behind the counter and stood beside me. Silently instructing me to watch, he took a small, bumpy rock between his fingers and very gently eased its two halves apart. I glimpsed something membranous in the opened-up space. Something was pulsing there and gradually moving outward. Finally two little living forms (not recognizable as any particular creature) pushed their way out onto the counter. I couldn't believe the man had done that! What's more, he was obviously showing *me* how to do it. I tried my hand at it, and before long, tiny creatures were running across the counter. Somehow I had learned how to release life from within these seemingly lifeless rocks. I was amazed and thrilled. The man pointed to two little ones and said, "You can take these with you." Maybe as a reminder that I really had been able to achieve what seemed a miraculous feat.

Reflecting on this dream, I realized that I already possessed the tools I needed to do my healing and bodhisattva work: my own two hands. But despite this vivid dream, I made no changes in my career plans. After all, I was on track for nursing school: I'd done all my pre-reqs, and becoming an RN would give me job security and a variety of options.... Besides, I was preparing to take my bodhisattva vows, spending most of my time studying the scriptures, meditating and doing my hospice volunteering. It didn't seem like the right time to be making other big life decisions — taking vows was a big enough commitment to prepare for.

Then, one day a few weeks after I'd taken my vows, in the middle of meditation, a thought rose up: "You don't need to do nursing. You have your hands." Around this time, I'd attended my first nursing school orientation. To tell the truth, by this time, I had my doubts about whether this was really the kind of work I wanted to do. You see, I wanted to be Florence Nightingale, sitting by patients' bedsides, tending to them with love, but nurses these days have precious little time to work that way. During my morning meditation I realized that Reiki was the best way to do the healing work that appealed to me. It reminded me of the man in my dream: he didn't need any special tools in order to ease the rocks open and let the life essence within them emerge — he did it with his hands alone.

I thought about how he had done this. The key to his technique seemed to be that he moved very slowly and silently and gently, with infinite care and love, and just opened the rock up so that whatever was inside could emerge. This was exactly the way I was striving to use Reiki: to give my undivided attention to each patient or client, bring them comfort, and facilitate whatever healing resulted. Buoyed by this insight, but not yet sure of whether I should actually change my life plans because of it, I called up the head of the nursing program and asked whether I could defer my acceptance for a year. The answer was no. So, I took a couple of days to think it over, then gave up my spot. And committed to making my combined Reiki and Buddhist practice the core of my life.

Over the next year, as my work with hospice patients intensified, as I went on to do my Level II and Master Level Reiki trainings and started up a private Reiki practice, I still did not stop to consider what exactly Usui Sensei had had in mind when teaching his students. I just blindly accepted what people always said about Reiki: it's a hands-on energy healing method developed in Japan in the 1920s by Mikao Usui. A Buddhist practitioner, Usui Sensei had an insight experience after a 21-day mountaintop meditation retreat, and as a result realized that he'd developed marvelous healing powers. He spent the rest of his life doing healing work and teaching his students to do the same. This has always been the standard explanation of how Reiki came about and what Usui Sensei's purpose was in teaching it. And I accepted that. I had no reason not to.... Except for what I'd begun to experience while practicing both Reiki and Buddhism.

❧

I'd decided to take the bodhisattva vows the year before I received Reiki training. Taking the vows didn't mean I had to become a Buddhist nun or live in a cloistered community. What it did require was a 24/7 commitment to cultivating my own ability to act for others' benefit. Part of that means strictly observing precepts such as not killing, stealing, lying, or drinking; not engaging in sexual misconduct, harsh speech or idle talk; not harboring ill will, and not withholding help from others. Another major piece of my practice was studying and meditating so as to gain a deep understanding of the way we shape our own reality through our actions.

But for those of us who study Tibetan Buddhism and aspire to do bodhisattva work, another key focus of our practice is cultivating and nurturing bodhicitta, that boundless love and compassion for other beings. Meditations that help cultivate bodhicitta form a key part of my Buddhist practice. When I mention this, my friends and clients often ask me, "How does one go about loving people?" What they really mean is, "How does one go about loving *everyone*, all the time, unconditionally?" This isn't something we are born knowing how to do. His Holiness the Dalai Lama has remarked on this many times. Thankfully, Buddhism provides many tools to awaken and nurture bodhicitta, and I make continual use of them.

It was while I was deeply focused on my Buddhist study and these meditations, in preparation for taking my vows, that I received my first level Reiki training and began working with the dying. I noticed right away that when I'd give Reiki to others, I would feel an upwelling of tenderness for them, even if I had just met them for the first time. Connecting with people through Reiki seemed to enable me to experience something akin to the love that would arise during my meditations.

This was very consistent – I would do Reiki, and not only would the recipients feel relaxed and happy as their pain and anxiety faded, but I would be filled with joy, too. Yet, at this early stage of my Reiki practice, I certainly did not consider that the joy and love I experienced from connecting to others through Reiki might be the *goal* of the practice. I was still thinking that we practice Reiki solely to give others the energy they can use to alleviate their physical pain or psychological or emotional distress. The joy *I* was experiencing seemed like little more than a nice side benefit for my own personal spiritual practice: I was grateful that Reiki dovetailed so beautifully with my Buddhist practice and seemed to enhance my spiritual growth by increasing my feelings of love and joy.

It was still a while before I realized that this joy was, in fact, the *key* to my spiritual development; that the main reason for giving Reiki was to elicit this joy, which I could then share with everyone around me — through Reiki and in my life in general — and which would facilitate healing in others. I can pinpoint the moment when this insight came to me.

I'd begun doing 3-days-in-a-row sessions for clients and friends, and a few of my Reiki friends and I wondered what it would be like to engage in this intensive work as a share: we would do group sessions on each other for three days straight. So, four of us who felt very comfortable with each other and had given Reiki together previously, began meeting once a month for these three-day shares: one of us would lie down on the table, and the other three would give her Reiki. Then we'd rotate, until everyone had received a short session. So, on each of these three days, we'd spend about two hours giving and receiving Reiki. Under these conditions, practicing with people we felt close to and comfortable with, we experienced a connection to each other and a joy deeper than we'd ever before felt during Reiki.

If you're a Reiki practitioner, maybe you've had occasion to feel that giving Reiki became like a meditation. As you rest your hands in one spot for a while, it can begin to feel like the body beneath your hands is part of you. This is a natural physiological process of losing the awareness of a boundary between your hands and what they're touching, the way you cease to feel the clothing on your body as you wear it. Even so, when giving Reiki becomes meditative, and when in your stillness you cease to feel two separate bodies, you can then become aware of just the presence of energy flowing unimpeded, just moving, as if not from or to any definable being. At the same time, you know that you are there with another human, and as you feel this energy connection, you feel closer to him or her, happier. You might feel a surge of joy and love.

This is precisely what my friends and I experienced during our first 3-day share. At one point, during the second day, one recipient wanted to lie on her side for her session. I was at her front, one of us was at her feet, the other at her back. The two of us at front and back had our arms draped across her side, each of us reaching over her, forming what she later said felt like a comforting cocoon. As we stood there, silently, I happened to glance down at her face, and was overcome with joy and tenderness. She looked just like an angel to me, and I felt so grateful at that moment, to be able to bring her this healing energy together with our other friends. I glanced at the one standing at her feet, and she smiled, and then at the friend across from me, and understood that she and I were feeling the same thing — there were tears in her eyes, too.

We talked about what had happened, that our Reiki share had somehow enabled us to feel deeply connected, and that joy and love arose when we felt that connection. But we also knew that we don't automatically feel this whenever we practice Reiki. I think that what made our experience possible is that we were all committed practitioners, knew each other well, had given each other Reiki often, and were all engaged in some kind of spiritual practice. What's more, we were in the middle of an intensive series of sessions. All of this came together in a way we had never experienced before with such intensity.

That is when I suddenly grasped what Usui Sensei meant by "happiness": the joy that arises from feeling so deeply connected to others that you can't help but devote the rest of your life to sharing that joy with others by treating them with love and working for their benefit. I believe Usui Sensei experienced this love, or bodhicitta during his mountaintop retreat, and that feeling the "happiness" he described led him to develop and spend the rest of his life teaching a system that could help his students experience ever stronger and stronger connections to each other, potentially even bodhicitta and the joy that arises along with it. In other words, Usui Sensei was teaching his students how to invite true and lasting happiness into their lives and spread this joy to everyone with whom they came in contact.

Even achieving the first true, fleeting experience of bodhicitta, as I believe Usui Sensei did during his retreat, is extraordinarily difficult. If we could get there by practicing a little meditation or Reiki here or there, everyone would have experienced it. Buddhist teachings stress how rare it is, even for extremely highly-trained, dedicated practitioners like Usui Sensei. An experience of bodhicitta may occur only after years-long practice, if ever.

Given the rarity of such an occurrence, it's no wonder that, as Buddhist teachings tell us, a profound experience of bodhicitta, even if it last only a few seconds or minutes, changes the way you view the world forever: it inspires you to go even more deeply into your spiritual practice, so that you can nurture your bodhicitta and help it grow by feeling this connection and joy again, thereby deepening your devotion to helping others. You work to experience this connection and joy and love over and over, for longer and longer periods of time, until finally, it does become a permanent state.

True bodhicitta is, of course, far deeper than what my friends and I experienced during our share. Even so, that day, when we received a faint hint of what this love might feel like, I was filled with gratitude toward Usui Sensei. He was a genius! Feeling my own excitement and seeing how inspired my friends also were by what had happened, I felt sure that this was what Usui Sensei had been striving to help his students discover.

How did Usui Sensei achieve this state of happiness in his own life? We don't know for sure, although we do know that he was a committed Buddhist practitioner. We're told that, following his mountain-top retreat, he suddenly acquired the ability to facilitate profound healing in others using the energy that flowed through his hands. But since we know that Usui Sensei was a serious, long-time Buddhist practitioner, we can describe his achievement another way: by devoting his life to cultivating compassion and insight, Usui Sensei gradually achieved a personal transformation so deep and rare that he was able to experience the boundless love Buddhism calls "bodhicitta." Certainly, those who encountered Usui Sensei afterwards would have sensed his boundless love for them and naturally experienced healing as a result.

Although Usui Sensei felt drawn to help others cultivate this same ability, he would also have known, from his own experience, that not just anyone can facilitate great healing simply by placing their hands on another person. After all, he was able to do this only after a profound transformation resulting from years of Buddhist practice. Usui Sensei would have known that not everyone could — or even wanted to — work toward such an experience by practicing Buddhism deeply, as he had. So he developed a system he could teach to laypeople. He found a way to offer his students a seemingly simple, yet powerful — and terribly challenging — way to progress spiritually without being monastics. Rather than committing to being monks or nuns, they could practice in the midst of their daily lives, going as deeply as they wanted in the pursuit of this happiness.

I believe that in order to develop the framework he taught his students, Usui Sensei took the Buddhist tools he had used in his own transformation, then modified them so he could teach them to anyone, whether they were Buddhists or not. I believe he knew that if he took students through this work, step by step, they, too, could experience transformation, great compassion, and deep, abiding happiness. Then they would also naturally acquire the ability to help others find healing.

❧

As I mentioned in the Introduction, once I understood through my own experience what I thought Usui Sensei was striving for, and had experienced deep transformation myself, I created the practice framework I offer in the book, so that I could help others use Reiki to transform their heart, mind and life. But how has my life changed since I began practicing in this way? I'll tell you a bit about that, so that you'll have an idea of what working in this way might do for you.

One of the first benefits I noticed was that my worries, insecurities and resentments began to fade. As they did, I started worrying less about trying to make sure people were getting results from their sessions with me and was able to put my energy instead into simply offering people Reiki with kindness and love. Once I shifted my focus to giving, I began to sense stronger connections during Reiki sessions than I ever had before. Not only were my clients getting more out of sessions, I began feeling great joy and tenderness toward them! Over time, it became easier and easier for me to work this way and establish a strong connection when giving Reiki.

As I began to feel this closeness consistently, my compassion and love for those around me gradually increased. I felt more and more joy. Don't think that my life became free of problems or disturbances. It didn't! But, buoyed by the happiness that arose from my practice, I grew able to deal with challenges more and more easily. What's more, because I was happier and less easily thrown off by difficulties, I grew kinder and more patient with those around me. My interactions with everyone around me gradually became more joyous, because they were infused with my own happiness. This was a marvelous feedback loop of feeling joy and tenderness arise and then sharing it with others. Every time I'd give another Reiki session, the whole cycle would begin again.

What I discovered, as my joint Reiki and Buddhist practice deepened, was how to start up this cycle of giving and receiving joy and then keep it going. By making Reiki and Buddhism my life's practice, I came to experience — and be able to share with others — a happiness far, far greater than I ever imagined was possible. Now I can't imagine living my life any other way!

To develop the framework I now teach to students, and which forms the core of *The Heart of Reiki*, I essentially worked backward: I asked myself, how was I able to get to this point? I secularized the Buddhist techniques that I'd brought into my own Reiki work, so that they'd fit into a non-Buddhist Reiki practice, while still offering practitioners comparable benefits. After all, my students, like Usui Sensei's, aren't necessarily Buddhist, and so I, too, wanted to present a practice that would work for all practitioners, no matter what their spiritual orientation, and no matter what level of training they've had.

How closely does the Heart of Reiki practice resemble what Usui Sensei taught his students? I can't say, but I certainly believe it is in the spirit of his teachings. And I have seen in myself and in my students that practicing this way allows us to reap the happiness that arises from our growing connection with others and transforms our lives. I invite you to explore this book. It is my hope that by devoting yourself to this practice, you, too, will begin to experience the happiness Usui Sensei intended, and share it with everyone around you, both through Reiki and in all other moments of your life. And so, I invite you to explore this book and this practice.

CHAPTER TWO

Is This Path For You?

There's no one personality type or life's circumstance or background that the Reiki practitioners who have found their way to this practice share. Even so, a common thread does link them: they're all looking for a calmer, happier life and more joyful connections with others. They want to find a way to not be swept away by their disturbing thoughts or emotions, and a way to treat those around them with more kindness.

These practitioners are all unique in terms of the difficulties they face, the negative habits they'd like to see fade, or the source of their unhappiness. Some people feel angry or sad a lot of the time. Others get tired out because they give so much without protecting their own time and energy; they want something that will sustain *them* for a change. Some simply feel unhappy and don't know why. Others feel a yearning to connect with a higher force, or God, or what they call their Soul, or to heal their mind and body and find their way out of whatever is holding them back in life. Some say that they feel their spiritual practice is missing something, or that they would like to develop a spiritual practice. They would like to transform their heart and mind so that they can be more loving to others and so that their negative emotions and life's ups and downs won't take such a toll on them.

In short, those who come to this practice feel drawn to engage in a process that will facilitate transformation and allow them to experience greater happiness in their lives and share that happiness with those around them. If that resonates with you, then perhaps this practice can help you set out on that path.

In Chapter One, I talked about how I have seen my life change since I've been practicing Reiki the way I'll teach you here. So, what might you expect to get out of the practice? I can't say for certain what transformations you will see if you enter into this work, but I can tell you about what my students have experienced as they've engaged in this practice.

A very real benefit they have noticed is that although they feel anger, they "manage not to get caught up in it" or in other negative feelings about themselves or others. Practicing has helped them gain this insight: "Just because I feel it doesn't mean I have to act on it." They are learning to choose not to act out of anger or other negative feelings: "Worries still come up, but I'm able to put them aside."

In terms of how the practice has benefited their interactions with others, one student told me, "People take me more seriously and treat me more respectfully now."

My students also note that they're getting more from the Reiki now. They say things like, "I find myself releasing things I didn't even know I was holding on to." One spoke of working with her partner as "a meeting of energy, a feeling of completeness." Another described doing the practice as "recycling the loving feelings" and reported that the "calmness that it gives me carries not just for the day, but for days."

Sometimes my students are at a loss to describe the way they are benefiting from this way of practicing, like the woman who described her experiences as "so profound that I can't find the words. "

Although students benefit in their own, individual way, the common thread is that as they engage in this practice sincerely and diligently, they begin to see positive change in their lives.

✤

By engaging wholeheartedly in this practice, especially if you are working with a partner, you will make it possible for your strongest negative emotions to fade, but without consciously trying to make that happen.

When giving Reiki, whether to ourselves or others, we may find ourselves focusing on results, even if it's only that we're looking to feel more relaxed after a session. When we work with clients or offer Reiki to our friends or family, it's hard not to hope for a benefit — after all, we give Reiki precisely because people generally feel good after receiving it.

But the way you'll use Reiki as part of this practice is all about *allowing* transformation to take place, instead of trying to *make* it happen. It's focusing on engaging in the practice itself that allows whatever transformation is ready to take place within your body, mind and spirit to play out.

Certainly, in order for the transformative shifts to occur, you will need to do the practice a certain way, but that is your only task: you'll follow the practice and observe what changes begin to take place. I'll explain this more in the practical section, but here's an example of how one of my students experienced this process:

As he practiced, this student began to find that it became much easier for him to notice when he was beginning to be angry. Once he was able to see his anger beginning to arise, he was also able to allow it to fade before it swept him away. As he has continued, he's found that he's grown less likely to feel anger in the first place. This is what the practice makes possible: you develop growing awareness of when disturbing thoughts or emotions are arising and also gain the ability to cope calmly with them.

In order to facilitate this transformation, you set aside thoughts about trying to *make* something happen, and put your effort into doing the energy practices/meditations and the self-Reiki and the hands-on and distant Reiki with a partner, and into bearing the Reiki precepts in mind. Then, something *does* happen. It's just that you're not *trying* to make it happen.

This is the beauty of this work, and the paradox: if you learn to focus on the actual ongoing process of carrying out the practice, you will see changes. That is the key: trust the practice and follow it as I will lay it out for you. *Just practice!* When I say *Just practice!* I mean for you to focus on the practice itself, not on what results you'll get from it.

The Heart of Reiki offers an approach to experiencing transformation that stresses consistent, active practice rather than logical thinking or reflection. If this appeals to you, then *The Heart of Reiki* will be a good fit for you. But before you turn to the next chapter and begin planning your journey, take some time to consider whether you've got a ready supply of the following provisions, all of which you'll need as you move along this path:

Sincerity: If you sincerely want to experience transformation and are eager to do the work that will help discomfort fade and happiness grow, then this practice will help you do that. Maybe you're thinking, What's the catch? Of course I want to experience transformation and be happier!

In Buddhism we talk about renunciation, which means being so sick of the suffering in your life that you want to learn how to free yourself of it. Your devotion to this practice doesn't have to be quite that dramatic, but the more motivated you are to invite happiness and calm into your life, the easier it will be for you to develop a strong practice.

Openness and Flexibility of Mind: I encourage my students to engage in the practice and see what happens. I don't mean that in a "watch the magician and see what happens" way. What I mean is you will get the most out of this process if you go into it *without* a certain goal or outcome in mind. That way, you are free to grow in whatever way becomes possible, not just in the ways you envision at the moment.

When I say "flexibility of mind", I'm talking about being willing to see yourself, those around you, and the world itself, in a new, more positive way, with less disturbance. This is exactly what the practice will help you do: gradually let go of your usual, upsetting way of seeing everyone and everything. This happens naturally as you relax and practice.

Discipline: If you make your practice a regular part of your life and schedule, and practice consistently, working with Reiki this way can lead to deeper transformation than you ever imagined possible. Think of it this way: call to mind the teacher or mentor or advisor who has meant the most to you in your life, who has given you the best advice — guidance which has helped you along in your work or personal life. Now imagine that this person offers to come spend as much time with you as you would like, answering your questions and mentoring you so you can excel at what you're doing. I bet you'd say, "Great! Come on over! Stay as long as you like!" It's the same with this path. The potential for growth is limitless if you devote time and energy to the practice. In the next chapter, I'll give you some hints about how to develop a routine you can stick to.

Patience: The key to experiencing positive shifts in your life is to keep working sincerely and to give the practice some time. You'll begin to see changes gradually: at some point you'll begin to notice that you've begun to see the people around you differently. Maybe you don't feel insulted when someone didn't appreciate you; maybe you won't explode angrily when someone pushed your buttons. Maybe you'll step outside one morning and think that somehow the world looks brighter or sharper. The first time this happens, you'll think, "Wow! Something really is happening here!" So, *Just practice*, and soon you'll notice the benefits of your practice beginning to arise.

Trust in me as your guide: If you decide to enter into this practice, you will be allowing me to lead you along an unfamiliar path. I developed this framework out of the methods I've used during my own transformative process, as I described in Chapter One. Since I've gone through many small and large releases of habitual ways of seeing those around me, I understand what that process can feel like and can explain to you how to use the practice to move through periods of turmoil and experience these releases yourself. In other words, since I know this road well, I can help you travel along it, too.

I take my role as your guide very seriously and thank you for your trust in me and these teachings. I offer this practice to you sincerely, hoping that you, too, will see greater and greater happiness enter your life as you practice.

Maybe now you have a sense of whether you feel drawn to step onto this path to happiness. In the next chapter I'll describe the practice elements and explain how to go about making them a regular part of your life.

Chapter Three

Preparing for Your Journey

Sometimes my friends or clients or students ask how I organize my own personal combined Reiki and Buddhist practice. Most often, it's because they know I meditate, and they think meditating might help them feel calmer and deal with life's stresses more easily. So they ask me how often I meditate, for how long, and so on. I tell them that right at the start, I decided I'd get up earlier every morning and meditate, no matter what; that I made it my first activity each day, instead of leaving it until later in the day when I might be tempted to put it off in favor or because of other pressing tasks.

When they hear that, people often shake their heads. Every day? Get up earlier? No way! I can't do that. I reply that in earlier years I never would have done that either. But finally, I got to a point in my life where I was so stressed out and disturbed and so sick of feeling that way that I decided to put the time I'd otherwise spend worrying to positive use in meditation!

That was the beginning of my practice. Over the years I have gone through periods of more intense practice, such as during the year when I was preparing to take my bodhisattva vows. Or in the winter of 2011, when my son was going through Marines Officer Candidates School, and I decided to make my own practice more challenging in solidarity with him as he was going through that rigorous training.

But no matter whether I am engaged in my usual routine of meditation, study, writing and Reiki practice, or in a period of more intense practice, what keeps everything running smoothly and enables benefits to keep arising in my life is consistency.

I mention this consistency and the positive effects that come from my own practice because acquaintances have asked whether I feel overly restricted by my very regular practice schedule. I reply that on the contrary, I find it liberating. Sticking to a consistent routine actually frees up a lot of time for me: because I regularly meditate at set times every morning and evening, I don't spend time twice a day deciding when to meditate. I *know* when I'll be meditating, so my mind is not distracted by extra decision-making.

When my son was doing his training, which involved sticking to a very precise schedule, I instituted a very strict regimen for myself, too: meditation time, writing time, eating times, times for seeing clients, walking time, etc. The first two weeks were tough, because I'd been used to deciding everything on the fly pretty much every day. But once I'd gotten used to the routine, I loved it! Because I knew what I was doing at each time of the day, I was able to focus better on each activity, without part of my mind thinking, okay, what are we going to do once we're done with this? All of that chatter settled down and I was able to concentrate on everything I was doing. I benefited so much from that set routine that once my son finished his training, I kept it more or less in place, because I felt so much more focused on what I was doing and was getting even more enjoyment from everything.

I mention all of this because developing a routine for yourself will make it so, so much easier for you to follow this practice. Rather than restricting you, a regular schedule will help you experience benefits more quickly.

So, first let's look at the elements that make up the Heart of Reiki practice framework. Then I'll give you some hints about how to set up a routine that will work.

Practice Elements

You'll do some of these elements every day, some once a week, some on an ongoing basis or once a month. I take you through them in detail in the next chapter, but this will give you a rough idea of what each of them entails.

Daily practice elements:

- **Doing Gassho:** Gassho is a Japanese term for putting your hands in front of your chest, palms together, in an act of gratitude and respect. We do this every day as we begin practice, and at the beginning of distant or hands-on Reiki practice.

- **Repeating Usui Sensei's precepts:** These phrases have come down to us from Usui Sensei and are inscribed on his memorial stone in Japan. They include his Reiki precepts, which guide us in choosing our actions every moment, as well as his explanation of what Reiki is, and his succinct instructions for how to use the five precepts. Reciting these words every day helps us remember why we are practicing:

> *The secret of inviting happiness through many blessings*
> *The spiritual medicine for all illness*
>
> *Just for today:*
> *Do not be angry*
> *Do not worry*
> *Express gratitude*
> *Devote yourself diligently to your work*
> *Be kind to people*
>
> *Do Gassho every morning and evening*
> *Keep the precepts in your mind and recite them*
> *To improve your body and mind*

- **Daily energy practice/meditation to increase your energy flow:** In each stage of our practice, I'll introduce you to a new energy practice/meditation. Doing these meditative exercises not only increases your awareness of energy flow in your body, but also helps you develop concentration and an ability to not be thrown off by distractions around you.

- **Daily self-Reiki:** Giving yourself Reiki every day is one of the foundations of your practice. But you'll be doing Reiki for yourself in a way that's probably different from how you learned to do it.

- **Reflection on one the Reiki precepts:** At each stage of your practice, you'll take some time to reflect on one of Usui Sensei's precepts, to consider how you might understand it, and how to integrate the precept into both your Reiki practice and your life as a whole.

Weekly or semi-weekly elements:

- **Reiki for animals or pets, if you have one:** You may not always have a person in your household who can serve as a volunteer Reiki recipient for you, but you may have pets, and giving them Reiki a few times a week will boost your practice, even though the animals are not giving you Reiki back!

- **Weekly distant Reiki for someone else, preferably as a trade with a partner:** This is the second element of your practice that involves working with another being, this time a human! You can do this even if you are a Reiki I practitioner and have not yet been formally trained in sending distant Reiki as part of a Reiki II class.

- **Weekly hands-on Reiki trade:** Do this as a two-way trade with your practice partner or another Reiki practitioner, or work with a volunteer who would like to receive Reiki on a regular basis.

- **Regular communication with a teacher, to discuss the practice and receive an attunement:** (*Optional*) Although you can go through this entire practice on your own, being in touch with a teacher who practices Reiki in this way can really help you move along your path. Questions will inevitably come up, and it's good to have someone to go to for answers and advice. Feel free to contact me, and you may have a teacher in your area, too, who might be interested in working with you on this practice, so do seek out opportunities for that kind of collaboration.

Another reason to consider working with a teacher is so that you will have the chance to receive regular attunements. Usui Sensei gave his students attunements frequently, not simply as an initiation associated with a given level of training, and you will also benefit from receiving additional attunements.

The Six Practice Stages

You may recall that that earlier on I urged you to step onto this path without looking for an outcome. Although this book does include six stages of practice, think of this as an ongoing practice, rather than a program to complete.

Since the transformation you will facilitate as you move through these stages has no natural ending point, the deeper you go into the practice, the more you will benefit. There is no limit to the happiness you can experience and invite into your life.

Moving From Stage to Stage

Even though there's no fixed end point to this practice, you will need to decide how quickly to move through the stages. When you begin working on Stage One Practice, and even as you move ahead to other stages, take your time. I say this because I am someone who for years always hurried through any program I thought might be useful. I wanted to learn everything, figure out how to do everything, and then do it! It was not until I began practicing both Buddhism and Reiki that I finally learned to work without rushing, and to focus on the practice instead of the result. So, with this practice, think process, not finish line.

Moving at a relaxed pace is particularly important when you're starting out, because you'll need time to get comfortable with the practice elements and develop a schedule. It may take even two or three weeks for you to feel that you've got the elements down, and that's okay. Give yourself that time. Enjoy it. After all, that's what this is all about: allowing happiness to arise by using Reiki in a new way.

As a general guideline, I would say that it would be good to spend a couple of months on each stage. More if you want. You gain nothing by rushing. In Chapter 5 ("Gauging Your Progress") I'll write in more detail about how to gauge when it's time to move on to Stage Two Practice. But for now, it's best to concentrate on setting up a schedule that will work for you and getting comfortable with the practice elements.

Establishing a Practice Routine

Now that you've decided that you want to do this practice, if you're at all like me, you will just want to get started, right now! I have always tended to jump right into things once I decide that's what I want to pursue. Speaking of this single-minded devotion to goals I've set for myself, my mother once said to me, "If you decide to do something, we'd all better just get out of your way. There's no stopping you!" She meant that in a positive way, but over the years I've learned that it's not a bad idea to make sure you've got all your gear before you head up Mt. Everest. Metaphorically speaking, of course. So, before you actually begin working on Stage One Practice, give yourself a little time to consider how you will fit the practice elements into your daily schedule.

Here are some ideas:

❋ **Daily practice elements**: Your daily routine will include doing gassho, reciting the precepts, doing the energy practice, and self-Reiki. Bundling them together works well, because you can move smoothly from one to the next, and they don't take too much time. About half an hour a day will do it, which works out to about fifteen minutes each for the energy meditation and the self-Reiki. Or spend longer on the self-Reiki. The more, the better! But as you're beginning your practice, set aside half an hour.

What time of day is best? I suggest starting your day with this practice, because once it's part of your routine, particularly if you get up half an hour early to do this, when all sane people are still happily abed, you'll have a better chance of making it happen every day. What's more, you'll be beginning every single day refreshed and focused and Reiki-ed!

But what if your household is populated by small beings who demand your attention in the early morning, as soon as they sense the slightest rustling of sheets in your bedroom? If you have little children or slightly older kids whom you see off or deliver to school, or dogs that just have to be fed and walked right at the crack of dawn, then trying to fit practice in right at that time might seem to be courting disaster. If this sounds like your life, then by all means, pick a different time of the day for practice, but make sure it is one that will work consistently. It might be 10 a.m. on Monday, Wednesday and Friday, and 2:00 p.m. on Tuesday and Thursday, and 3:00 p.m. on weekends. Some people like doing the practice right before bed, because then they can just go to sleep. But for others, by the time it gets to the end of the day, they're exhausted, so they end up skipping practice. What's key is to pick times that are doable for you and then commit to them.

Speaking of others in your household: when you are ready to start doing this practice, let them know that you're starting new Reiki work that includes some daily exercises. Let them know that this is important to you, and that you would love it if they'd support you by being understanding when it is your practice time. Tell them (nicely, of course!) that it will help you so much if they don't knock on the door or play loud music or choose your practice period as the time to drill the holes in the wall to hang up the new flat screen TV. If they're skeptical, tell them it's likely that doing all of this will mean you will be calmer and less stressed out, which will be good for them, too!

One caveat: although I have had my set practice periods for years now, there are times when I do adjust the schedule. When my kids have had performances or special events, when we have out-of-town visitors, and so on, I do not make a big deal about sticking to the schedule at all costs. That doesn't mean I skip practice; I just pick a different time during the day, because although keeping my practice up is paramount for me, I also want to be considerate of those close to me and support them in *their* important endeavors.

But when you are starting out, work extra hard to set and keep to your schedule. Before long, you'll be so used to it that if for some reason you shift it one day, everyone in the house will say, "Hey, isn't it your Reiki time?" That's the way it should be.

✳ **Weekly practice elements:** In addition to your daily practice, you'll be giving distant Reiki and hands-on Reiki once a week, and giving Reiki for an animal approximately three times a week.

As you did with your own individual practice, set a regular time to trade Reiki with your partner. This can take a bit of work at first. I've been trading Reiki weekly with my best Reiki friend for several years now. When we first started working together, we'd schedule week to week. Each time we met, we'd open our calendars and say, "When's good for you next week?" This was just a crazy way to go about it, because sometimes we'd find it hard to identify a time when we were both free. That meant we were in danger of missing our precious Reiki time. Yikes! So, finally we picked one morning as our dedicated meeting time and entered it in our calendars for every week at the same time. Sometimes we adjust it forward or backward half an hour or so, but we've been able to keep it going for all this time precisely because we're committed to not scheduling anything else during that time.

That's what I encourage you to do, too: pick a time with your partner that will generally work for both of you and *pen* it in to your calendars, bearing in mind that you will probably need to adjust it every now and then. But at least you won't risk missing practice entirely.

How about working with animals or your pets? Am I really going to ask you to schedule a set time for giving Reiki to your pooch? No. In the next chapter, I'll give you some ideas about choosing a time to do animal Reiki, but this can be much more flexible, and you can take your cues more from the animals, as long as you do consistently find time to give them Reiki.

Finding a Practice Partner

How do you go about finding a practice partner? For that matter, what are you even looking for in a partner? (I do want to say, that if you can't find a practice partner right away, definitely go ahead and begin working on the elements you can do on your own. When the time is right, the pieces will fall into place, and you will find someone to work with.)

First of all, bear in mind that the person you work with does not have to be doing *The Heart of Reiki* practice, too. They just need to be willing to do the weekly hands-on and distant trade. Once they hear you talk about the practice and experience the difference it makes in how the Reiki they receive from you feels, though, don't be surprised if they want to join in, too.

Here are some ways to identify possible candidates:

- The first place to look is among your Reiki-trained friends and acquaintances. If you received your Reiki training in a class with other students, ask whether any of them would be interested in trading distant and/or hands-on Reiki with you on a weekly basis, assuming you enjoyed being with them in class, of course!

- Attend a Reiki share in your area. If your Reiki teacher doesn't hold Reiki shares, ask whether he or she knows of any in your area. Once you find one, talk to others who attend. Many folks who attend Reiki shares are eager to find more opportunities to give and receive Reiki.

- Talk to your Reiki teacher. Let him or her know that you're starting this new practice and are looking for someone to work with. He or she might be able to connect you with like-minded students and will probably also have a sense of which of those students might be a good fit for you. Failing that, your teacher probably knows other teachers, and they might be able to introduce you one of their students.

- Talk to Reiki teachers, including your own. Reiki teachers are regular folks, too, and maybe your teacher — or someone else's — would jump at the chance to take his or her Reiki practice deeper by working with you. You'll never know unless you ask!

Speaking of fit: How can you judge whether someone would be a good practice partner for you?

There definitely needs to be a certain amount of compatibility between you and your practice partner: if you're going to be trading hands-on Reiki with someone every week, it should be someone you like at least a little! A person you feel relaxed with. You need to be able to count on him or her to show up for practice and not cancel at the last minute or call up every week, asking to change the time because something has come up. You will probably be able to tell very quickly whether or not a given person will work as a partner on an on-going basis. If you begin working with them, but then realize this is someone who annoys you or is not reliable, then don't hesitate to thank them kindly and find a new partner!

Having said this, I also want to encourage you not to have too many preconceptions about who might be a good fit for you. Someone who at first seems unlikely might turn out to be a fabulous partner. For example, when I began teaching this practice, two students who had met each other before, and had even attended my Reiki shares together began working together. Although I never would have thought to pair them up as partners, they ended up complementing each other very well and found it easy and enjoyable to work together.

So, as you are looking for a potential practice partner, don't be too quick to count someone out. I suggest that if you are considering working together, get together and trade hands-on sessions, and see how you both feel about it. If you aren't comfortable with that person, then look for someone else to practice with.

What if you talk to all the Reiki practitioners and teachers you know, and you still can't find anyone to work with?

Just because you can't line up someone to work with right away, doesn't mean you won't find a partner later on. Also, it's important to remember, as I said earlier, that working alone is not a hindrance.

Even though doing the practice without a partner means that you will not be *receiving* distant or hands-on Reiki from another person, what's most important is to have someone to whom *you* can give Reiki every week. So, go ahead and recruit a volunteer. It can be the same person every week or a variety of people, but I suggest lining up a couple of people to give Reiki to regularly so that you are not spending lots of time each week trying to line up volunteers. Think of friends or family members to whom you'd enjoy sending Reiki, and ask whether they'd be willing to have you do that for them. Tell them that you're doing a new Reiki practice and that the program involves distant Reiki and hands-on practice once a week.

Finding a Teacher to Work With

As I've noted earlier, you can certainly work through the entire Heart of Reiki practice on your own. But having access to a teacher who can guide you is a real benefit. So, if you think your Reiki teacher would be interested in serving as a resource for you as you practice, don't hesitate to approach him or her. Or, you could ask your Reiki-trained acquaintances whether they think their teacher might enjoy helping you with the practice. It's worth asking around, and consulting with a teacher or two.

Once you find a teacher who's interested in working with you, it's important that he or she feel positive about the practice framework, so that you'll both receive as much benefit as possible.

So, now you're ready....

Now that you've taken the time to prepare yourself for your journey, turn the page and enjoy getting started with Stage One Practice.

CHAPTER FOUR

Stage One Practice: "Just for Today, Do Not Be Angry"

As you step onto this new path, I invite you to reflect briefly on what brought you to this practice. I can't say how you ended up here, but I'll bet *you* can. So, take a few minutes now to sit quietly and ask yourself: Why am I beginning this practice? What benefits am I hoping to see in my life? Either simply reflect on these questions, or actually write down your thoughts. If you prefer, make some notes about this at the back of the book, where you'll find blank pages just for that purpose. This will help you later on, when you're trying to gauge the benefits of the practice. So, take three, five, ten, twenty or more minutes now to reflect. Then come back and get acquainted with the elements of your new practice.

Now that you have some ideas about why you're beginning this practice and how you'd like to see your life change, set them aside. You don't need to think about them in order to benefit from what you're doing. It's true that some of the practice elements, such as reflecting on the precepts, will involve conscious reflection. By and large, though, it's by committing time and sincere effort to this practice that you'll gradually begin to see benefits in your life. Simply devoting yourself to the practice has a way of targeting the areas of your life that can most use transformation at the moment, even without your ever making a conscious decision to address them. So, as you begin, *Just practice!* and see what happens. When I say that, I mean to focus diligently and consistently devote time and sincere effort to this work, because that's how using this practice will invite happiness into your life.

Stage One Practice: Here is a quick summary of the elements that make up the first stage, some of which you'll do every day, some once a week, some on an ongoing basis or once a month:

- Doing Gassho, followed by repeating Usui Sensei's Reiki precepts (keep your list of precepts handy until you memorize them.)

- Daily energy practice/meditation to increase your energy flow.

- Daily self-Reiki.

- Throughout Stage One Practice: Reflection on the first Reiki precept: "Just for today, do not be angry."

- Reiki for a pet three times per week.

- Weekly distant Reiki with a partner, if you have one, or for someone else of your choosing.

- Weekly hands-on Reiki with a partner, if you have one, or for someone else of your choosing.

- Optional: monthly communication with a teacher, to discuss the practice and to receive an attunement.

Note: The Appendix at the end of the book contains a brief summary of all the practice elements for each stage. You can use it as a quick reference to review the elements as you're learning them.

Stage One Practice, Step by Step

First day of practice

Start by setting aside half an hour when you will not feel rushed and, ideally, when you will not have to jump up and race off somewhere afterwards. I recommend doing this part of your practice first thing in the morning, because it helps you start off your day calm and focused, but any time of day can work, as long as you strive for consistency. Commit to a set time each day to do the practice. Choose choose different times on different days if you need to, but make it a regular part of your schedule. During the first few days, it's particularly important to give yourself the time to settle into practice, to focus on what you're doing with a minimum of distractions.

Find a spot in your room, apartment or house where you can sit without being interrupted. (If you live with others, let them know that this is your practice time and ask them politely not to interrupt you unless it's an emergency!) You don't need to make a big ritual out of this by surrounding yourself with special items or incense or talismans. It's not about that. It's about finding a quiet, comfortable space where you can practice without being distracted.

Make the space as serene as possible — no TV, no radio, no music, no computers, no cell phones, even on vibrate! If you have a land line phone, either turn off the ringer, or put it in another room under a pillow so you won't hear it if it rings. Turn everything off and put your phone and computer where you will not be tempted to look at them! If you have pets, choose a practice space where they won't be able to bother you, if that's possible. Wear comfortable clothing. In short, do everything so that you won't be distracted.

Sit wherever and however you want — on a chair, on a couch, on the floor, on a meditation cushion — as long as you are comfortable but not in a position where you're likely to fall asleep!

Once you're settled in to your space, you're ready to begin your daily practice.

Here's how:

Each day, begin by doing the following:

✠ Gassho and expressing gratitude

We begin our practice each day by putting our hands in front of our chest, palms together, a position the Japanese call "Gassho". This is a common gesture in Japan, and it indicates both respect and gratitude. Put your hands in Gassho, close your eyes, and give thanks that you have the opportunity to do this practice that will benefit both you and others.

Next, while keeping your hands in Gassho, recite aloud the following phrases written by Usui Sensei. View this recitation as a way to sincerely offer your gratitude for having the opportunity, time and motivation to be doing this practice that has so much potential for benefitting you and those around you, to remind yourself of the purpose of this practice, and to set your intention to have ongoing awareness of the precepts Usui Sensei taught. Give your full attention to the words as you slowly repeat them:

The secret of inviting happiness through many blessings
The spiritual medicine for all illness

Just for today:
Do not be angry
Do not worry
Express gratitude
Devote yourself diligently to your work
Be kind to people

Do Gassho every morning and evening
Repeat the precepts and keep them in your mind and heart
To improve your body and mind

What Usui Sensei means by "do Gassho" is to put your hands in Gassho and then bow from the waist, to show thanks and respect to your teacher, fellow practitioners, and the teachings. So, once you've done this recitation, do Gassho again.

Type up these words and print them out (or write them out by hand) so you'll have them handy until you've memorized them.

- **Daily energy practice/meditation** (10 minutes at first, then build up to 15)

In each stage of practice, I'll introduce you to a new energy practice/meditation that will help you learn to focus your attention and also increase the energy flow through your body. This first exercise involves visualizing the energy in your body flowing into and out of a spot in your abdomen, which in Japanese is referred to as the *hara* or the lower *dan tien*. We can translate this as the "elixir field," the spot in the body where our life force is stored. It's located about three finger widths below the navel.

Why focus on moving energy (which we can refer to as "ki," the same "ki" as in "Reiki") into and out of the hara? Long-time karate practitioner and teacher Jeffrey Brooks explained it to me this way: "It is easy for people to learn to generate energy from the hara because that is the ocean of energy at the center of the body. That is where we first breathed from as an infant, and it is the strongest pool of ki in a healthy body. The breath and body and mind are united there, and the energy can easily flow from there along any meridian or channel in our body or through the body of another person."

The exercises I present here are, in fact, a kind of meditation. You do them in silence, devoting your full attention to visualizing the energy moving. Doing these exercises not only increases your awareness of energy flow in your body, but also helps you develop concentration and an ability not to be thrown off by distractions around you.

Do this energy practice/meditation each day after you recite the Reiki precepts.

Here's how:

First: Sit with your spine and neck as straight as possible. (Although your spine and neck should be straight, don't strive to have your legs at a 90 degree angle to your back. A 135 degree angle, where your knees are slightly lower than your hips, is preferable, since it puts much less strain on your lower back. If you're sitting on a chair or couch, just sit so that you can lean back very slightly.) Put your hands in your lap, with the back of your left hand resting atop the palm of your right hand. Closing your eyes may help you to concentrate.

Start with a few slow breaths in and out, while focusing on relaxing your shoulders and jaw. Allow your breath to flow in and out at the pace that feels most natural to you. Take care to exhale fully before inhaling again.

Once you feel that you are relaxing and breathing easily, imagine that as you inhale, energy flows into you and down through the central channel of your body, all the way into the middle of your abdomen, your hara. As you imagine the energy moving down into the hara, think of it like a stream of water flowing slowly into a vessel and gradually filling it. Inhale and imagine energy flowing into your hara. There's no need to force it — just visualize it naturally moving into that vessel. As you exhale, simply be aware of the vessel there. Allow the energy that has flowed into it to rest there. Repeat this cycle of breathing and pulling energy into your hara.

On the first few days, do this energy practice for five to ten minutes. Then work up to fifteen minutes a day. Move from this energy practice right into...

�֎ Daily self-Reiki session (20 minutes)

Giving yourself twenty minutes of Reiki every day is one of the keys to keeping your energy moving. Besides, it simply feels great! The ideal time for a session is right after you finish the energy practice/meditation, because you are already in a relaxed, receptive state and in a suitable physical setting. I think you'll be pleasantly surprised at how easy it is to move into Reiki after doing the energy practice.

You were probably taught to do self-Reiki when you did your Level I training. In case you weren't, I'll give you a few suggestions below. But even if you are used to doing Reiki for yourself, as part of this practice, you'll be working differently from the way you've been taught before. Often, when we sit down to do Reiki for ourselves, it's because we have an ache or pain, or because we're upset for some reason. We think, Oh! I can make myself feel better if I give myself Reiki! But for our practice, it's most important to approach the self-Reiki without looking for results. Your goal is not to try to bring about healing; it is simply to allow the energy to flow through you and leave it at that. *Just practice.*

Here's how:

Let's assume you're doing your session right after the energy practice/meditation. (If you've chosen a different time, be sure to find a comfortable position in a quiet space where you won't be disturbed, using the guidelines I've given you up previously.)

- Remain seated as you were. A good way to start is to close your eyes, take a couple of breaths in and out and ask yourself where you feel drawn to put your hands. If a certain part of your body seems to be calling for attention, just put your hands there and let the Reiki flow. Maybe you have an ache or an upsetting thought that's been bothering you, and it's fine to bear that in mind as you choose a hand position. But don't overthink it. Pick a spot and go with it. Once you decide where to put your hands, forget about the reason you put them there. Rest your hands in that spot and just give yourself Reiki. Leave your hands in that spot as long as you want.

If you feel moved to shift your hands to another position, go ahead, but just let the energy flow without placing expectations on yourself or the energy. The fewer hand positions you use, the better, because resting your hands in one or two positions for the entire session will help you go more deeply into the Reiki.

If you feel yourself slipping into checking how you're feeling, or wondering what you could do to help yourself feel better, try doing the energy practice from above while you give yourself Reiki. It will help you concentrate on just letting the energy flow, rather than on results.

- Continue for about 10 minutes the first few days. Gradually work up to twenty minutes of self-Reiki every day.

- If you find yourself becoming very distracted, it's okay to put on a little instrumental music to listen to as you give yourself Reiki, but working without music will help you go more deeply into the Reiki, so I suggest you consider trying that.

✻ Reflection on the first Reiki precept: Just for today, do not be angry

At each stage of your practice, you'll take some time to reflect on one of Usui Sensei's precepts, consider its meaning, and think about how to integrate your understanding of the precept into both your Reiki practice and our life as a whole. But before asking you to turn your attention to the first precept, I want to talk about the precepts as a group and what I believe Usui Sensei had in mind in teaching them.

Mikao Usui's Five Precepts

When you first heard or saw the five precepts, they may have reminded you, as they did me, of the Ten Commandments or the precepts that Buddhist practitioners observe. Like these, Usui Sensei's precepts are words to live by. Yet Usui Sensei was not teaching his students Buddhism. He was offering them a practice method which, although inspired by Buddhist teachings, was suitable for anyone, no matter what their spiritual beliefs. I am sure he did not intend for the people he taught to accept the precepts as religious dogma, as articles of faith. Rather, I'm sure he hoped the precepts would inspire his students to engage sincerely in the practice.

To me it seems crucial that Usui Sensei told his students to bear recite the precepts and keep them in their mind and heart, just the way one might recite prayers or a mantra. He didn't give his students specific instructions about *how* not to be angry, or worry, or how precisely to go about being grateful and diligent and kind. He just had them recite the precepts. Of course he would have hoped that the precepts would inspire his students to take care with their actions, thoughts and speech. But he also would have known, from his own Buddhist practice that committing to precepts does not magically make it possible to live them. He would have known that if you want your disturbing emotions to fade so that the virtues of gratitude, devotion and kindness can arise in their stead, you need to do two things: you need to both make a commitment to live according to virtuous principles *and* devote yourself to a practice that both brings tranquility and makes insight possible. This is what monks or nuns do in any spiritual community. They state their commitment to an ethical life by taking vows, and they observe a rigorous practice framework which both helps them keep those vows and makes it possible for them to gain deep spiritual insights.

Now, although Usui Sensei was teaching laypeople, not monks and nuns, it seems clear that he based his own work with students on these same principles: he gave them basic guidelines for how to live and taught them a practice that would help them keep to those standards of behavior. Although he was not teaching within a monastic setting, and his students were not taking formal vows, I imagine he wanted a way to help his students affirm their commitment to the ethical life the practice was helping them live out. So, instructing them to recite the precepts every day seems to me like a lay equivalent of having them take vows. Buddhist teachings stress the importance of taking vows and explain that actions we take in accordance with vows are much more powerful in their effect than those we take under regular circumstances, without a previously stated commitment. Usui Sensei would certainly have been aware of this, and I believe that encouraging students to recite the precepts daily was his way of offering them the chance to commit to their practice in a way that resembles the commitment a spiritual practitioner makes by taking formal religious vows.

Thus, I see Usui Sensei's precepts both as a set of goals to which students commit to aspire, as well as a description of what they *can* achieve if they engage wholeheartedly in their practice. It's as if, by presenting the precepts, Usui Sensei was saying to his students: practice the way I teach you, and this is what will happen. Commit to the precepts and pay attention to what you say and do and think, because you do have control over that. Also put your focus on *just practicing*, because that is what will transform your mind in the long run and make it easier and easier for you to observe those precepts, thereby inviting happiness into your life.

This is precisely the way you will work with the precepts as part of your Heart of Reiki practice: you'll keep the precepts in your mind and heart as you practice, to remind yourself of what you're shooting for, and to strive to bring them to bear as you choose what to do or say in your daily life.

Although Usui Sensei presented his precepts in a specific order, that doesn't mean he intended for you to work only on not being angry and then, once you perfect that, to move on to not worrying. He instructed us to repeat *all* the precepts every morning and evening, and to keep them in our mind and heart. So, he must have intended for us to bear each of them in mind as much as we could, at all times. Even so, I've chosen to focus on one precept at each stage of this practice. This will allow you to both recite all of the precepts every day and go more deeply into one of them at a time. During Stage One, then, you will place a bit more focus on not being angry.

Working with the first precept:
"Just for today, do not be angry."

You don't need to start this part of the practice on your first day, if it seems like too much to begin the self-Reiki, energy practice and this part all at one time. But don't wait too long, either, because all of the elements work together and reinforce each other. Give yourself a couple of days to settle into your practice, then set aside about twenty minutes the next day, at a time when you can sit and give the precept your full attention. This is an important element of your ongoing work, because the reflection you do now sets the foundation for increasing your awareness throughout your work at this stage. So, don't rush through it.

✳

Have you ever wondered by Usui Sensei began his precepts with "do not be angry"? I think he placed not being angry and not worrying at the top of the list because these two powerful disturbing emotions make it difficult for us to feel grateful, or devote ourselves to our work, or to be kind. Thus, although Usui Sensei doesn't tell us to wait to engage in the last three precepts until we're free of anger or worry, I believe he felt that using our practice to help anger and worry fade would naturally help us observe the last three precepts, too. So, let's take a closer look at the first precept.

Let's start by asking why Usui Sensei might have encouraged us not to be angry, instead of just blindly accepting the precept. This is a key step, because if you're not convinced that anger is something you're better off without, then you won't be as motivated to continue with this practice that can reduce your anger.

To begin, take a sheet of paper (or use the blank pages in the back of the book) and note down some situations in which you have reacted with anger in the course of your daily life. Be as specific or as general as you want. For example: "I yelled at the kids when they made a mess in the kitchen," or "I was so mad at my boss for falsely accusing me," or "I got really mad when people weren't listening to me," or "I lashed out when I felt disappointed." I'm sure you can come up with at least a few examples of situations like these. (Note that I'm not asking you to say you won't react with anger in such cases, only to brainstorm and be aware of what some of them are.)

I'm sure any of us can easily recall times in our lives when we've gotten angry. But what about if you're a Reiki practitioner? Has anger ever come up as you were practicing Reiki? That might seem unlikely at first. After all, we associate giving Reiki with happiness and comfort. Really, have you ever ended up yelling at someone during or after a Reiki session? I doubt it! Even so, anger and annoyance *can* arise. Maybe we're doing Reiki for a friend or family member with whom we've recently had a disagreement; or we've reluctantly agreed to give someone Reiki at an inconvenient time and we're feeling a little taken advantage of; or a client was late to a session, or even didn't show up. In any of these cases, annoyance or anger can arise.

These emotions can also take more subtle forms during or after a session. Let's say the recipient doesn't seem to experience any immediate benefit: his knee still hurts after receiving Reiki, or she is still depressed about a breakup, or even seems more upset than before the Reiki. Or, he's new to Reiki and had the nerve to sit up after the session, shrug, and say, "I didn't feel a thing." Because these people have not responded to Reiki as we'd hoped they would, we may get annoyed — at them or at ourselves.

If we've felt this kind of annoyance and even anger, does that mean we are awful Reiki practitioners? No. It means that we are not immune to anger just because we practice Reiki.

So, now that you've come up with some examples of times when you've become angry, think about the consequences of anger in your life: when you react angrily to people, how does it affect them? How does it affect you? If you have trouble answering these questions, recall the last time you got really angry and reflect on that incident.

Next, go ahead and consider how your life might be different if you felt less anger. What might be possible for you if anger was not clouding your mind or prompting you to react negatively to those around you? How might you or others benefit? You can just mull this over, or use the blank pages at the back of the book to make notes.

As you were thinking about this, perhaps it occurred to you that allowing anger to fade in your mind might make it easier for you to observe Usui Sensei's other precepts: if you're less angry, you'll be able to act with more kindness toward others or feel more grateful for what is going well in your life. Even if you didn't add this to your list, I'm sure you came up with a number of ways your life would be different if you experienced less anger, and how those around you would also benefit from having less anger in the air. I imagine you do feel that you'd be better off if you could avoid angry outbursts and feelings. But *how* can you manage to not be angry?

Usui Sensei's instructions explain exactly what to do: "Repeat the precepts and keep them in your mind and heart." And practice diligently. Focus on your practice instead of your anger and let your sincere, consistent practice do the work.

But what to do when you do feel anger rising up within you? In such cases, your practice will help you ride anger out without being swept away by it. Silently repeat, "Just for today, do not be angry," when you find yourself beginning to feel angry. Repeat it to yourself silently like a mantra, over and over, distracting your mind with it until the anger or annoyance fade. You can even start out saying, as one of my students did, "just for right now", and then work up to "just for today." *Just for right now, do not be angry.*

Giving yourself Reiki can also help keep your anger from growing once it appears. If you begin to feel angry, try to find a place to sit for a few minutes and give yourself Reiki. Reciting the precept at the same time will help your mind focus on something other than the person or situation that's angering you. If the anger persists, set aside some time later in the day to give yourself a longer Reiki session.

One more way to help anger subside instead of letting it out is to devote five or ten minutes to the energy practice/meditation. This allows you to focus on something besides your anger, and it also helps the energy move to your hara so that you'll begin to feel more stabilized and calm.

By using your practice this way, you're not pushing anger down or away. Rather, the practice elements are helping you remain calm in the face of the disturbance, making it possible for you to ride out the turmoil until it fades on its own, which it will. The key is to remember to use the practice elements when you begin to feel upset. The more you practice this, the easier it will become for you to recognize anger when it's just beginning to arise, and you'll be able to turn quickly to the precept, self-Reiki or the energy practice/meditation. Chapter Six, "Using Your Practice to Survive Turmoil," will teach you more about using your practice elements when you're upset.

Once you have done this reflection about the first precept, you don't need to repeat the process. Reciting the precepts each day — in a focused way that reaffirms your commitment — will serve as a reminder to you that anger is one of the negative emotions from which this work will help free you. Put your energy into the practice, not thought *about* the practice.

❈

The elements I've just described are all for you to do on your own. They don't require participation from any other beings! The next three parts involve working with others. This regular Reiki exchange with others, whether human or not, is a key part of this practice. It accelerates the transformative process for both partners.

❊ Reiki for a pet three times per week (10 minutes)

We may not always have a person in our household who can serve as a Reiki volunteer for us, but many of us do have pets, and giving them Reiki regularly will boost our practice, even though the animals are not giving us Reiki back! If you do not have pets, or don't have access to animals you'd be able to work on regularly, set aside this part of the practice for now and return to it if and when the opportunity presents itself.

Although you can give Reiki to your pets as frequently as you want, I suggest three, ten minute sessions a week so that it becomes a consistent part of your practice schedule.

You may already be giving Reiki to the animals in your life, but, as with the Self-Reiki, you'll approach the work differently now. Even though your dog may have arthritis, or your cat is old and her teeth might hurt, when you sit down to do Reiki for them as part of your practice, set all of that aside. You don't need to figure out where they hurt, or wonder whether the Reiki is easing their pain or discomfort. Does that seem cold-hearted? It's quite the opposite! Practicing this way will allow you to connect more deeply with your pet, without being distracted by a desire to accomplish something during the session. I think you'll find they'll get even more from the Reiki this way. Just put your hands on them and let the energy flow. *Just practice.*

Here's how:

I recommend giving your pets Reiki at a time when they are already resting comfortably. Otherwise, if you do the sessions when they seem to be in pain, you might slip into wanting to use the Reiki to help them feel better and be distracted from focusing on your practice. You can even do it while they're sleeping. I'll take you through doing the practice on a cat, but you can easily adapt this to other types of animals (although you may not want to try putting a horse in your lap...)

Sit down next to your cat, or put him on your lap, if that is convenient, and lay your hands on any spot you wish. If you know he has a painful place on his body, go ahead and put your hands there if you want. Otherwise, any spot that feels right to you is fine. Focus your attention on allowing energy to flow into the animal, and once you feel you have established that connection, forget about trying to do anything else. Leave your hands on that spot for ten minutes, or fewer, if your cat decides he's had enough and gets up and walks away.

As you're doing the Reiki, maybe your hands will feel warm or tingly, or you'll receive intuitive information about how the animal feels, or his pain level. Perhaps a visualization will come to you. Let all of that pass right through your mind without acting on it. Leave your hands where they are, no matter what information you're picking up. Your job is to bring the energy to the animal and nothing else. *Just practice.* When the ten minutes are up, pet your cat for a bit as thanks for helping you practice.

You can do Reiki this way for any animal in your life. If your pet does not tolerate hands-on Reiki, it may be that the energy just feels too intense, so feel free to start with a very brief session. Indeed, I think it often seems odd to animals when you first do Reiki for them. The first time I put my hands on my border collie's shoulders to give him Reiki, he seemed to frown. He turned his head to look at me, as if asking, What the heck is that? But before long, he lay his head back down, and after about a minute, let out a big sigh. Three minutes later, he was fast asleep.

Similarly, my cats, who were used to having me pet them, seemed surprised the first time I put my hands on them and just held my hands there, without moving. They seemed to be thinking, Hey, this isn't petting! One of my students told me that he's taken to informing his cat which "modality" he's using. He'll say, "Okay, that was petting modality. Now we're moving to Reiki."

Don't be surprised if your animals seem a little confused by Reiki at first. But don't give up! A way to ease them into this new mode of communication is to give them Reiki the first time by holding your hands just above the body. And always let them end the session whenever they want. If they get up and walk away, don't be insulted or discouraged; it probably just means they've taken in as much energy as they need.

As you make this a consistent part of your practice routine, I am sure it will be a joy for both of you, a regular way for you to connect and enjoy each other's company.

Now let's see how to integrate working with other humans into the Heart of Reiki practice, in two ways.

�֎ Weekly distant Reiki for someone else, preferably as a trade with a partner (20 minutes)

This is the second element of our practice that involves another being, this time a person! You can do this even if you have not yet been formally trained to do so: I'll explain how to go about it below. First I'll go through how to work with a partner. Then I'll explain how you can do the practice even if you do not yet have a partner.

Working with a partner:

Although your partner needs to be Reiki trained, he or she doesn't necessarily need to be doing this practice, too. He or she can do distant Reiki according to his or her training.

To begin, agree on a time once a week when you will send distant Reiki to each other, preferably the same time each week. Doing so will help build a consistent routine, so that you don't have to worry about checking in with each other to pick a time each week. Of course, schedules can vary and life's events can intrude, but do your utmost to keep to the time you pick. That way, you'll also have fewer occasions to use "Just for today, do not be angry" as your mantra. Some of my students even call each other right before practice time, just to check in, which makes it much less likely that one of them will forget!

You and your partner will take turns giving each other distant Reiki for twenty minutes each. Agree beforehand who will receive first.

Just as when you do self-Reiki, find a space where you can sit quietly without being disturbed during the session. You should be in a comfortable position, but not so comfortable that you'll fall asleep! Turn off all computers, TVs, radios, CD players, and silence your phone, unless you'll use it as a timer for the session. (But make sure you set it to ring only when the alarm goes off!) Working in silence is best.

Doing the distant session:

- Before you start, do Gassho, then spend a couple of minutes doing the first half of the energy practice/meditation, to get your own energy flowing.

- Sit comfortably and imagine that your partner is lying in front of you the way he or she would be if lying on a Reiki table in front of you, but that his or her body is the size of a stuffed animal, about 12 to 14 inches long. (You can use an actual stuffed animal as a surrogate for the session and put your hands on its crown.) Close your eyes and call to mind your partner. See him or her in your mind's eye and imagine that his or her entire body is present before you. Think his or her name to yourself if you wish, then focus your attention on simply being present with him or her and connected through Reiki. If you haven't been formally trained in sending distant

Reiki, don't worry. As long as you have the intention for the Reiki energy to go from yourself to your partner, it will. If you do not yet feel energy flowing through your hands, focus on moving energy into your arms from your hara and out through your hands until you feel that they're energized.

- Put your hands in the spot where you imagine the crown of the person's head to be. Leave your hands there for ten minutes. Then imagine that you are now positioned at your partner's side, and place your hands where you imagine the hara to be. Leave your hands there for ten more minutes.

- Just as you do when doing Reiki for yourself or your pet, focus on sending the energy without trying to figure out what your partner needs or whether the Reiki is having an effect. Just establish the connection and send the Reiki. No matter what imagery or intuitive information you receive, work only at those two spots. Your job now isn't to try to figure out what is going on with your partner; it's to establish as strong and stable a connection as you can and just send the energy along without being distracted by thoughts about what is going on in the body.

If you do find yourself becoming distracted, whether by your own thoughts, or by intuitive information you're picking up, do the energy practice/meditation while you're sending Reiki: keep your hands in the same position and continue giving distant Reiki, and at the same time visualize the energy flowing into your hara and collecting there. Your partner will still receive the Reiki just fine, and doing this can help you remain more focused.

- When you finish sending Reiki to your partner, do Gassho and settle back to enjoy receiving the Reiki your partner will send! Once you've completed both halves of the session, state your gratitude for having the opportunity to do this practice and do Gassho once more.

What if you don't have a partner to trade distant Reiki sessions with?

Even though working without a partner means that you will not be receiving distant Reiki in return from another person, you can still give distant Reiki to someone, and it will still benefit you. Think of a friend or family member to whom you'd enjoy sending Reiki, and ask whether they'd be willing to have you do that for them. Tell them that you're doing a new Reiki practice and that the program involves sending distant Reiki to someone once a week.

What about scheduling? You could pick a regular time that's convenient for you to send the Reiki each week and let the recipient know when that will be, so he or she can be on the lookout for it, or even make time to sit down and take advantage of the session. Or, the two of you can agree on a time that is convenient for both of you so that the recipient will have a better chance of being able to relax while you're sending the Reiki. Whichever way you do it, the main thing is to be consistent about doing this practice every week, even if your recipient's schedule changes. After all, although part of the purpose of doing this is for the recipient to receive the Reiki, the main point is for you to have the practice connecting with a recipient and sending the Reiki consistently, without giving in to distractions.

Do the actual distant Reiki session just the way I described above, even though you will not be receiving in turn.

✠ Weekly hands-on Reiki for someone else, preferably as a trade with a partner (20 minutes)

The last weekly element of Stage One Practice is for you and your partner to do twenty minutes of hands-on Reiki for each other. Once again, working with a partner who's also doing the practice is ideal, but not a requirement: you will do the session as I teach it here, and your partner will use his or her own method. Until you do begin working with a partner, do twenty minutes of Reiki for a willing volunteer. (See below for details on this.)

Where should you do this weekly share? If either of you has an office space with a Reiki table, do your sessions there. Otherwise, it's fine to meet at one of your homes: find a quiet room to work in where you're not likely to be disturbed. You can do the actual sessions either on a Reiki table or as chair sessions. Or the recipient can lie on a couch or across the foot of a bed, as long as the giver can find a way to be comfortable while working. (When I began doing a lot of Reiki with patient in hospitals and hospice settings, I bought a camp stool that is just the right height for bedside Reiki. You could also sit on a footstool if your recipient is lying on a bed or couch.)

So, you've found a comfortable space to work in, you've set up either a chair or a place to lie down, and you've made the place quiet by turning off TVs and radios, turning off the ringer on the house phone, silencing cell phones and asking any other household members to please not interrupt you, because you'll be doing your Reiki practice. Ahhhh… Now you can finally begin!

Your approach for this hands-on Reiki will be similar to when you do Reiki for yourself and your pets, or distant Reiki, in the sense that you will not be focusing on picking up intuitive information or figuring out where your partner needs Reiki, or on facilitating healing. During these sessions, you'll rest your hands on only two spots. At the same time, you will be doing a variation on the first stage energy practice meditation I taught you earlier.

As you work, you may well sense that this or that area of your partner's body is calling out for Reiki, or feel the desire to move to a different spot. You may even feel that you're not doing what you should to help your partner, the way you would in a typical Reiki session. If thoughts like these come into your mind, just let them flow on out again without acting on them. Remind yourself that this is not a healing session per se. This hands-on energy work is one element of the self-transformation or spiritual practice that you are doing with your partner. You are learning to work in a new way that will enable you both to use Reiki to connect more easily and deeply with each other and, eventually, with everyone to whom you give Reiki.

Doing the hands-on session:

- Begin your time with your partner by doing Gassho, reciting Usui Sensei's five Reiki precepts out loud together, and expressing your gratitude for the opportunity to do this practice with each other. Then spend 10-15 minutes doing the energy practice/meditation together before beginning your Reiki trade.

- Now, whoever will receive Reiki first can lie down (or take a seat, if you're doing this as a chair session.) Make your recipient as comfortable as possible — blankets, pillows, bolsters under the knees are all fine. Although it's easiest to do the practice if the recipient lies on his or her back, lying on the side also works. At this stage of practice, the recipient doesn't need to do anything other than close the eyes, relax, and invite the energy in!

- To begin the session, stand or sit at the recipient's head and do Gassho, to express thanks to your partner for allowing you to share Reiki with him or her. It's also a good way to physically indicate that you are beginning the session; it helps focus your attention. We all have our own way of connecting with a recipient when we're giving Reiki. For this practice, keep it simple: silently focusing your attention on the recipient is enough.

- Once you feel the energy begin to move through you, begin the energy practice/meditation: as you inhale, pull energy down into your lungs and then lower, into your hara. But now, as you exhale, imagine that you are sending that energy out of your hara, up into and down your arms, then out through your hands into your partner. Pull energy into the hara as you inhale and then send it out to your partner as you exhale. Take your time and to allow the energy to flow without forcing it. Just breathe at a natural, comfortable pace, and visualize the energy flowing gently in and out. This may feel awkward at first, but soon you'll settle into a nice, easy rhythm.

- With your hands in this position, give Reiki for ten minutes. If this becomes physically uncomfortable for you, shift your hands *slightly*, since you will find it hard to concentrate on giving your partner Reiki if you're in great discomfort yourself. However, do your best not to move once you put your hands down. Take care to position your own body so that you will be as comfortable as possible giving Reiki. Then you'll be less likely to experience discomfort.

- After ten minutes, one at a time, to your partner's hara: position your hand roughly between the top of the hipbones, with either your thumb or little finger (depending on which side you're standing on) just below the navel. Lay your hands in a line or one on top of the other. Rest them there and continue doing the energy practice/meditation as you send Reiki for another ten minutes.

- After you've given Reiki at that spot for ten minutes, remove your hands from your partner's body and do three sweeps: without touching the body, position your hands a few inches above the crown of the head and move them slowly down the center of the body, all the way to the feet. Come back to the crown and move your hands down either the left or right side of the body, then repeat a third time with the other side. This is a good way to mark the end of the session. It also smooths out the energy and keeps it from staying pooled in one spot.

- Do Gassho toward your partner and then lay your hand on his or her shoulder and tell him or her the session is over.

- Take a few minutes for your partner to have a drink of water, and then switch recipients. During this time, it's good to talk as little as possible, so as not to distract from the flow of the energy.

- When you've completed both sessions, do Gassho toward each other and express your thanks for the opportunity to work with each other.

What if you don't have a partner to trade hands-on Reiki sessions with?

Although it is ideal for you to have a fellow Reiki practitioner as practice partner so that you are both giving and receiving Reiki each time, the most important thing is to have someone to practice on every week. So go ahead and recruit a willing volunteer. It can be the same person every week or a variety of people, but I suggest lining up a couple of people to work with regularly so that you are not spending lots of time each week trying to line up volunteers. (See "How To Go About Finding a Practice Partner" in the previous chapter for some hints about this.)

Once you've arranged for someone to work with, carry out the session as you would if you were doing a two-way trade session, including doing Gassho at the beginning and end of the session, but without the

15 minutes of energy practice/meditation. At the end, thank the recipient for giving you the opportunity to do your practice with him or her.

✵ Monthly instruction, attunements and discussion with a teacher (Optional)

I have laid out this practice so that you can work through it on your own, because I really want you to be able to follow this path even if you don't have the opportunity to be guided through the practice by a teacher. However, you'll benefit greatly to work with a teacher, either regularly or occasionally, either in person or via phone or e-mail. I suggest this because I know from my own experience, and from working with my students, that questions and concerns come up, and it can make a world of difference to have a teacher to turn to. In addition, if you're working on your own, you might wonder about whether you're doing the practice correctly, or whether it's time to move to the next stage.

Here's how I work with my students. (This is a model you could follow if you're working with a teacher.) I meet with my local students — either individually or in a group, if the students are all at the same practice stage — once a month to discuss how they're doing with the various elements, answer questions, introduce them to new energy practice/meditations if they're ready to move ahead, discuss one of the precepts, do hands-on Reiki with them, and give them attunements. The attunements are an important part of working with my students. They re-establish a strong energy connection between us, which the students say gives them a boost, both in terms of energy flow and mood. If they feel they are at a plateau in their practice, the attunements get them jump-started again!

This monthly meeting gives me a good sense of what benefits the students are receiving and what they're finding challenging, and I have the opportunity to give them support and encouragement and adjust the practice elements for them based on what they're experiencing. Students will occasionally come in feeling that they are doing something the wrong way, or that what they are experiencing is not what they *should* be experiencing, so our meetings are a time when I can reassure them and help them relax about the practice. Within the Buddhist tradition, a group of practitioners is called a *sangha*, and this is how I think of myself and my students: we support and encourage each other in a practice that is not necessarily easy to maintain on our own, simply because very few people are doing a practice like this!

So, I strongly encourage you to work with a Reiki teacher in some way, so that you will feel that you are being supported and encouraged on your path, and so that your questions don't go unanswered.

In the next chapter, "Gauging Your Progress," I'll help you judge what benefits your practice is bringing you, and explain how to decide when to move on to Stage Two.

CHAPTER FIVE

Gauging Your Progress

Once you've gotten comfortable with Stage One Practice, settled into a routine and have been practicing for a few weeks or a month or so, it's good to reflect on what positive effects you're seeing from practicing. That's what this chapter is all about: helping you recognize the benefits that your practice is bringing you and helping you decide when to move on to Stage Two Practice.

Identifying the benefits you're receiving

You can be sure you're on the right track with your practice if you are experiencing some of the following:

- You find that your ability to focus during the energy practice/ meditation and the Reiki sessions has increased.

- It has become easier for you to do the energy practice meditation.

- You are more aware of the energy flowing through your body.

- You are less distracted while giving or receiving Reiki.

- You feel you are going more deeply into the session when you receive Reiki.

- People who receive Reiki from you tell you that it feels deeper, or that it feels like you're working on a different level, or they are experiencing more or deeper releases during and after sessions.

- Your reflection on the precept has helped you see incidents in your life differently, even just once or twice.

- You are feeling more patient with yourself, others, and the practice.

- You are feeling happier.

- You feel little resistance to keeping to your routine.

- The practice was very challenging at first, but you've persevered and settled into a consistent practice.

- You feel a sense of accomplishment at meeting those challenges.

- You find that it's easier to settle into activities, both during practice and in other areas of your life.

- You feel you've learned some new skills which are helping you in your life and your Reiki practice.

- You feel more committed to the practice.

Noticing some of these benefits in your life is a sign that you are practicing effectively. The more of these positive results you're seeing, the more effective your practice is. Keep doing what you're doing!

No matter how strong your practice is, certain aspects of it might seem challenging to you. Here are some possible challenges and suggestions for working through them:

- *You sincerely want to do this work, the practice elements seem doable to you and you feel you're doing a good job at them, but you have a hard time setting up or sticking to a schedule.* This is the most common reason practice doesn't come together for people — their lives are so busy that they find it hard to make a schedule and stick to it. If this is the case, then working harder to stay in the routine can give your practice the boost you need.

Enter your practice times into your calendar, either on paper or in a smart phone, if you use one. If you commit to setting aside specific times to practice, then you won't double book yourself. The key is making the commitment to finding space in your schedule for this.

What if you've done this, but find you still are not practicing regularly? Take a good, hard look at what's coming between you and your routine. If others in your household are taking your attention at those times, then let them know that your practice is really important to you and ask them politely to honor those times.

Focus on getting your routine down. Once you do, it'll be much easier to keep going, and that's when you'll also begin to experience the deep benefits the practice can bring.

✤

You've set up a consistent practice schedule, and you've stuck to it, but you think you should be seeing greater benefits by now. If you've managed to overcome the obstacle of scheduling, you're probably very disciplined and are committed to your practice. That's a major achievement! You may actually be so committed that you are super anxious to experience results, maybe even impatient. This can make it hard for you to relax and approach the work as a process, to allow yourself to be guided by the idea of "see what happens."

The key here is to strike a balance between staying focused and being relaxed and flexible enough that you will be open to experiencing whatever the practice brings your way. The Buddhists express this idea by talking about a guitar string: if you tune it too tightly, it will snap without making any music, but if you don't tighten it enough, it will be too slack to produce a single note. It's the same with this practice: you need the discipline to keep practicing every day, but the patience to approach it without anxiously waiting for that note to sound.

✤

Really, what all of this comes down to, is that you want to experience transformation and benefits from this practice. You will! Trust yourself and the process and give it a little time, and positive results will definitely arise. So, keep at it and ... *Just practice!*

When's the right time to move to Stage Two Practice?

The first thing to remember is that there's no rush. You could do the first stage of practice for the rest of your life and continue to benefit from it. However, adjusting your practice slightly by moving to the next stage can increase the positive effects you'll see and facilitate more transformation — assuming you've laid a good practice foundation in your Stage One practice.

So, how can you tell if you're ready?

Here are some questions that can help you judge whether it's time to take that step, or whether you should stay at Stage One for a bit longer. When you can honestly answer yes to all of them, that's a great time to move to Stage Two:

- Have you set up a regular practice routine, and have you been following it faithfully for at least a month?

- Are you doing Gassho and reciting the precepts every day?

- Are you doing the energy practice/meditation every day?

- When you do the energy practice/meditation, does it come naturally and flow easily, or do you find that you need to re-read the instructions every time you do it? (You should move on only when you feel very comfortable with this part of the practice, since it is the cornerstone of all the variations that come.)

- Are you giving yourself Reiki every day?

- Do you feel that you're gaining some insight into the first precept, "Just for today, do not be angry" and have begun to notice when anger crops up in your life?

- Have you been doing Reiki regularly for a pet, if you have one?

- Have you been practicing distant Reiki once a week?

- Have you been giving hands-on Reiki once a week?

- Have you grown accustomed to practicing distant and hands-on Reiki the way I teach you, and have you begun to experience some benefit from working this way?

- Have you noticed some of the benefits that I mentioned earlier?

- Are you feeling confident about your practice and would like added challenge?

- Are you enjoying the practice?

Do you find this last question amusing? I ask this because it's always good to remember that the whole reason you're doing this practice is to help you invite happiness into your life. What's most important is to move on to Stage Two Practice only once you're feeling really stable with the Stage One. Otherwise, you'll be building the rest of your practice on a shaky foundation, which will hinder you, even in the short run.

So, take a good look at how your practice is going right now. You're the best judge of when to move to the next stage. If you're excited about moving on and learning some new variations on these elements, then go right on ahead.

More happiness awaits.

Chapter Six

Using Your Practice To Survive Turmoil

Now that you've been using your new practice for a while, I'll bet it's a little easier for you to sail through minor disturbances without getting as upset as you might have done before. That means you've already begun inviting happiness into your life! You've opened the door a crack so that it can begin to flow in. But consciously using your practice to meet more difficult challenges will throw the door open wider, so that happiness can stream in more strongly. Learning to do this is not just a handy benefit of your practice. It is, in fact, the *main* point of this practice. In this chapter, I'll teach you to do just that.

I grew up in northern Illinois, in tornado country. This is the way I remember my childhood summers: the sky would darken with storm clouds and the winds would come up. We'd check the TV or radio, and if they'd announced a tornado warning, we'd take refuge in the basement and ride out the storm in that safe space, coming back out only when the danger was past and the sky had cleared.

Similarly, in the course of our daily lives, emotional storm clouds or even tornados can come upon us, either with or without advance warning. Just as my family would ride out atmospheric disturbances by taking cover in the basement, you can use your practice elements more intensively to ride out emotional storms and emerge from them to see a fresh, clear horizon.

In this chapter, I'll give you tips for recognizing when an emotional storm front might be heading your way; tell you what you might experience as a full scale tornado is passing through; and explain how to use your practice elements more intensively to ride out the tornado. That way, instead of being buried under a pile of emotional rubble and debris, you'll be able to emerge unscathed.

Your personal refuge plan may vary a little, depending on the conditions, so let's look at how to work both with minor storms and full-blown tornados:

Dealing with a building storm front:

Back in Illinois, we always looked for a greenish sky and darkening clouds. If the atmosphere felt eerily still but still infused with tension, that was a warning sign, too. Here are some of the indicators that an *emotional* storm is brewing, whether inside you or around you:

- You might begin to experience a strong negative emotion, or feel irritated, antsy or anxious, without being able to identify anyone or any incident which set it off. You may be sitting quietly or lying in bed and suddenly you feel like you just cannot get comfortable, and the feeling persists no matter how much you change positions.

- Along with this emotional discomfort, or separately from it, you may feel unexplained muscle tension or pain in an area of your body where you haven't had an injury. You may feel this in parts of your body where you tend to store tension, or elsewhere.

Although you might not be feeling highly distressed when you begin to experience these sensations, they often signal that a larger emotional storm could be bearing down on you. If you hunker down and take cover with your practice *now*, instead of waiting until you're feeling more upset, your discomfort might fade without escalating into a full-blown tornado.

Here's how:

When you are still feeling only slightly uncomfortable, the best thing to do is to spend more time doing self-Reiki. In addition to your regularly-scheduled practice times, do 10-15 minutes (or even more) of self-Reiki each time you begin to feel the disturbing emotions or physical sensations. Remember to give yourself Reiki the same way you always do — without trying to make anything happen. By devoting your attention simply to giving yourself Reiki, you will both bring soothing energy into your body and distract your mind from focusing on the pain or negative feelings themselves. Before long, you will probably find that you're feeling much more comfortable.

This happens partly because the Reiki really does soothe and relax you. But what's more, the feelings that are distressing you naturally rise and fall in a cycle. You'll see, as you go through this cycle a couple of times, that the feelings generally start out mild, then get stronger and then eventually fade away. But we rarely notice the fading part of the cycle, because we often don't have the patience to just sit there in the middle of discomfort. We tend to want to run away from it or do something to get rid of it. But by sitting quietly with your discomfort as you give yourself Reiki, you're not only allowing that discomfort to fade: you're also beginning to form the habit of tolerating uncomfortable sensations, instead of being distracted and disturbed and trying to do something to dispel them. This ability to maintain your focus and not be distracted is precisely what you've been learning while practicing. Now you're able to use these skills to remain calm in the midst of a storm.

What's important is to actually *remember* to give yourself extra Reiki when you begin to be upset or uncomfortable. I can't tell you how often my Reiki friends, students and clients have been really upset about something, and when I ask whether they've been doing Reiki for themselves, they stop and think and say, "Oh. No, I haven't. I didn't think to do that." So, although we have this marvelous way to soothe ourselves right at our fingertips, it won't help us unless we use it. So, do!

Now, no matter how good you might get at running for cover when the sky darkens, there will still be times when you find yourself in the midst of a swirling emotional tornado. That's definitely happened to me! Sometimes these destabilizing whirlwinds seem to blow in out of nowhere. Let's look at what you might experience in such cases, and how using your practice will help you emerge even happier than before the clouds rolled in:

Recognizing and surviving the instant tornado:

> You might suddenly experience strong anger, sadness, jealousy, worry or anxiety in response to something someone does or says, or to a situation or place in which you find yourself. Sometimes your feelings are so strong that their intensity surprises you, or they are far stronger than the situation would seem to warrant. You may even think, "Wow! Why did that upset me so much?"

> You might feel yourself moving from feeling antsy or irritated to

a more intense discomfort. This can happen even if you've been doing more Reiki for yourself. You may become so physically or emotionally uncomfortable, that it could seem to you that there is absolutely no way out of these feelings or out of any situation that seemed to bring them on.

✠ You may despair, and feel you are lost, that everything is utterly hopeless and that you might as well just give up and accept your awful state. Maybe you will cry or feel like screaming or be really angry.

✠ You may fear your discomfort will never end and be horrified at the thought of feeling like this forever. You may feel like a caged animal.

✠ You may have a growing sense that you really need to take action to resolve the situation, because you think this will help you get rid of the discomfort. You might decide that nothing will get better unless you act, and that the time to act is *now!*

If you experience any of these states, then you are right in the middle of a full-blown emotional tornado. At this point, when the winds are strongest and you fear you're about to be blown away, you may feel you just can't take it. You can reach this point very quickly, in a matter of minutes or hours. Your only task at this point is not to try to stop the tornado, but rather to take cover.

Perhaps there are things in your life that you really do need to change, but you can't do that very well if you're in a panic. When you're feeling that way, it's best to take refuge in your practice, hunker down and keep yourself safe and comfortable until it passes, the way my family took refuge in our basement to ride out a storm.

Here's how:

✠ First of all, trust the practice. Trust that if you just keep practicing, the emotional turmoil and suffering you're experiencing *will* fade.

All the skills you've been honing since you began your practice will help you now in this very challenging situation. Working through the practice, you've gotten better at letting go of your desire to make things different. It's grown easier to maintain your focus despite whatever your body and mind are telling you. Using these same skills now will help you as you're faced with overpoweringly upsetting emotions.

✼ Go with the flow. When you're so uncomfortable, it's natural to feel that you want to do *something* to bring resolution. But what will help most at this point is to do your best to allow the discomfort to be there without trying to resolve or change anything. Tolerating the discomfort and allowing yourself to ride out the entire cycle of rising and fading negative emotions will actually help you get to the point where you'll feel your disturbance fade, and see relief and happiness replace it. It will happen on its own if you can just hold tight.

Is this easy? Not at all. Just coexisting with this uncomfortable state can feel like it requires great strength of will and conscious practice, because this is an unfamiliar way of approaching emotional turmoil. Really, most of us have little tolerance or patience in these circumstances: when we begin to feel tension or pain or anxiety beginning to build, we run to distract ourselves with anything that will dull our senses and our pain, or we get angry or scared and take some action we'll regret later on because it was taken in a state of disturbance. Just being aware of our desire to escape when we're feeling this way can make it easier to turn to our practice instead.

Another way you use your practice when you're feeling the urge to act on the messages you're getting from your body and mind is to...

✼ Distract yourself with *self-soothing*. This is your only job as you're moving through a major disturbance — to calm and comfort yourself. Your practice elements can help you with this. Do Reiki for yourself, for hours at a time, if that will help you remain calm. Ask your partner to send you distant Reiki or give you hands-on Reiki. Do your energy practice/meditation twice a day or more. When you're in the middle of this emotional upheaval, your body will probably feel very tense, so doing the energy practice will not only distract you, but also keep the energy flowing instead of locked in one place. Reflect on the Reiki precept that seems most relevant to your situation, or repeat one or all of the precepts as a mantra, over and over and over again. In short, trust the practice to soothe and calm you.

✠ Just because I urged you to go with the flow, it doesn't mean I'm saying you shouldn't do anything to try to alleviate your discomfort. On the contrary. In addition to stepping up your practice, take some ibuprofen, or a hot bath, meditate or listen to calming music. All of that will help you by helping you relax.

If you are experiencing great pain in your body, and it is really worrying you, then by all means, go to the doctor and make sure nothing is physically wrong. If you're extremely upset or anxious, then definitely check in with a therapist. Or call a friend, talk to a close family member, or ask your Reiki partner to help you by listening. Make use of your personal support network. Use any of these resources to help you make your way, but stick with the process. You can do it! And in addition to whatever else you're doing to remain calm, remember to keep up with your practice.

✠ Do Gassho and give thanks for having the opportunity to practice moving through this emotional tornado with focus and calm. Express your openness to that.

✠ Tell your teacher you're in a difficult situation and ask for his or her help. You may think that talking with your teacher is the very last thing you'd want to do when you're in the middle of this process. Maybe you think you'd feel embarrassed or not want to appear weak or vulnerable or idiotic or... But this is the time to transcend all of those doubts and make that phone call, because your teacher understands this transformative process, can help you recognize what is going on, and be a great support to you.

In fact, it can be a relief to talk with your teacher. I've found that my students often totally forget that their practice can help them get through an emotional crisis. So when I suggest they go more deeply into Reiki instead of putting it aside, they're actually relieved to remember that they have powerful self-help tools right at their fingertips. Similarly, your teacher can also encourage you as you ride the shift out and remind you that if you stick with your practice and ride it out, you will soon see the tornado fade in the distance. So, definitely, turn to your teacher for help. He or she will be so glad to support you in your transformation!

Just practice! I can't say it enough: when you're experiencing emotional turmoil, this is the time to practice more, not less. Keeping to your practice schedule and even stepping it up several notches will help you get through whatever is passing through. Let the practice help you!

Believe it or not, as you persevere through the tension and uncomfortable feelings you experience in the midst of a full-blown tornado, there will come a moment when all your distress will suddenly lift and you'll feel the relief and happiness that signals that the storm has cleared. It will feel as though the great discomfort you've been enduring for so long has suddenly melted away, leaving you happy and free of anxiety. If you've been feeling physical pain or tightness during the process, the release of that tension sometimes comes later, but you'll be surprised to find that it often just mysteriously vanishes. When you emerge from the storm cellar of your intensified practice, it will be like coming out of a house into the fresh, clear air after a storm has passed through.

The first time you experience this, you'll be amazed that you managed to get to a state of such happiness by not doing anything except sitting tight and engaging in your practice. This was an incredible revelation to me when I first went through it. Once I realized that throwing myself into my practice would bring relief and joy if I persevered, I began turning to my practice more and more — not just when a tornado blew in, but as soon as I sensed the first signs in the air. If you stick it out long enough, you *will* feel things shift to a place of calm and relief.

This is the heart of how your ongoing practice benefits you: it helps you develop the skills that enable you to move through life's most challenging situations with less and less disturbance. You see, by taking refuge in your practice and letting it help you stay calm, you're establishing the habit of remaining calm in the face of the most challenging situations in your life. That's what gradually reduces your suffering and invites more and more happiness into your life.

So, keep practicing, and although the tornado warnings will continue to sound in your life, you'll be able to use them as a way to strengthen your practice and invite more and more happiness into your life.

CHAPTER SEVEN

Stage Two Practice: "Just for Today, Do Not Worry"

Welcome to Stage Two! In this stage, aside from working with a new precept, you'll be learning variations on the elements you already know. This will keep you moving along smoothly in your practice.

You'll find a list of all the elements here, as a summary for you, with an asterisk after those that have new variations for this stage, plus full instructions for each element, even the ones that aren't new.

So, let's look at your Stage Two practice:

Stage Two Practice:

- Daily Gassho, followed by repeating Usui Sensei's Reiki precepts.

- Daily energy practice/meditation.*

- Daily self-Reiki.*

- Reflection on the second Reiki precept: "Just for today, do not worry."*

- Reiki for a pet three times per week.*

- Weekly distant Reiki with a partner, if you have one, or for someone else of your choosing.*

- Weekly hands-on Reiki with a partner, if you have one, or for someone else of your choosing.*

- Optional: monthly communication with a teacher, to discuss the practice and receive an attunement.

Stage Two Practice, Step by Step

Begin each day with:

- Gassho, expressing gratitude, and repeating Usui Sensei's precepts.

Put your hands in the Gassho position (with your hands in front of your chest, palms together,) close your eyes, and give thanks that you have the opportunity to do this practice that will benefit both you and others.

Next, while keeping your hands in Gassho, recite aloud the following phrases written by Usui Sensei. View this recitation as a way to sincerely offer your gratitude for having the opportunity, time and motivation to be doing this practice that has so much potential for benefitting you and those around you, to remind yourself of the purpose of this practice, and to set your intention to have ongoing awareness of the precepts Usui Sensei taught. Give your full attention to the words as you slowly repeat them:

The secret of inviting happiness through many blessings
The spiritual medicine for all illness

Just for today:
Do not be angry
Do not worry
Express gratitude
Devote yourself diligently to your work
Be kind to people

Do Gassho every morning and evening
Repeat the precepts and keep them in your mind and heart
To improve your body and mind

Once you've done this recitation, do Gassho again. Then proceed to...

- **Daily energy practice/ meditation** (15 minutes)

As in Stage One, do this energy practice/meditation each day after you recite the Reiki precepts. You already know how to do it: it's the energy practice you've been doing during the hands-on practice for Stage One. But now this new variant is your Stage Two energy practice/ meditation.

Doing the Stage Two energy practice/meditation:

First: Begin by doing the Stage One energy practice/meditation for a few minutes, until you have settled nicely into the cycle of drawing energy down into your hara as you inhale.

Next: Inhale in the same way as above, imagining that you are pouring energy into the vessel at your hara. But now, as you exhale, imagine that some of that energy moves outward from your hara in every direction, out of your body through every cell and pore of your body. Let the energy flow down into the hara as you inhale, then outward as you exhale. Again, there is no need to force it. Just visualize it flowing out, gently and naturally. Continue this cycle of breathing for a few minutes.

Continue practicing this way for 15 minutes.

Move from this energy practice right into…

✠ **Daily self-Reiki session** (20 minutes)

- Close your eyes, take a couple of breaths in and out ,and ask yourself where you feel drawn to put your hands. If a certain part of your body seems to be calling for attention, just put your hands there and let the Reiki flow. Once you decide where to put your hands, forget about the reason you put them there. Rest your hands in that spot and just give yourself Reiki.

Leave your hands in that spot as long as you want.

If you feel moved to shift your hands to another position, go ahead, but just let the energy flow without placing expectations on yourself or the energy. There's nothing you *should* be feeling during self-Reiki, so let go of that expectation, too!

If you feel yourself slipping into checking how you're feeling, and wondering what you could do to help yourself feel better, try doing the Stage Two energy practice you've just learned while you give yourself Reiki.

- Give yourself Reiki for twenty minutes every day.

✠ **Reflection on the Second Reiki Precept**: Just for today, do not worry.

We'll start by taking a look at what place worrying occupies in your mind and your life. I am not asking you to devote conscious effort to not worrying. Rather, you are simply exploring what form worrying takes for you. Then you will file away any insight you gain and shift back to devoting your time and energy to the practice. Remember, the practice will do the work, if you let it.

To start, think about the last few times you've found yourself worrying. Take a sheet of paper (or use the blank pages in the back of the book) and note down some situations in which you have felt worried. You can be as specific or as general as you want: "I was worried I'd lose my job," or "I was afraid Ellen would have a car accident in the snow," or "I worried about getting sick after a patient coughed in my face." Once you've made this list, consider whether these were isolated occurrences, or whether you regularly find yourself worrying in similar circumstances or situations. This can help you gain insight into whether you have patterns of worry tied to certain incidents, times of day, and so on.

Now let's think about how worry crops up when you're practicing Reiki. Can you recall any incidents when you've felt anxiety or worry while you were giving someone or yourself Reiki? Worry or anxiety *can* be part of giving Reiki. I used to worry quite a bit when I first began practicing Reiki. I'd worry that I was doing it "wrong". Were my hand positions right? Did I stay too long or not enough at a spot? Did my client smell garlic from my dinner on my breath? If clients came in great pain or suffering, I'd worry that they wouldn't find relief from the session. Afterwards, if clients made no comment, I'd worry that maybe they hadn't enjoyed the session. In short, although I always thoroughly enjoyed giving Reiki, an undercurrent of worry sometimes flowed beneath the surface in the early months of my practice.

Your Reiki-related worries may or may not resemble mine. So, take a few minutes now to consider whether worry plays any role in your Reiki practice.

Next, think about how you express your worry. Do you keep it inside, push it aside, talk to others about it, get angry, sad? Writing your ideas about this on a sheet of paper (or in the back of the book) can help you think this through.

The next step is to examine how your worrying affects you and those around you. Of course, worrying itself is a disturbing mind state, but ask yourself whether you or others experience negative results when you are feeling worried. If you have trouble coming up with an answer to this, call to mind the last time you were worrying about something. Try to remember how you and others reacted.

How could your life be different if you worried less? What might you be able to do that you're not able to do now because you worry? How could you, your friends and family benefit? Consider that question for a bit. As you're doing so, also think about how worrying less might help you observe Usui Sensei's other precepts, too.

�֍

Now that you've gotten a sense of how worrying affects you, and have considered the possible benefits of worrying less, let's take another look at Usui Sensei's second precept: "Just for today, do not worry." *How* do we do that? The same way you set about bringing the first precept into your life and Reiki work. You didn't consciously try to stop anger from arising. Rather, you poured your energy into the practice. That's what you'll do now, too. You won't start your day vowing not to worry, or go into a Reiki session *telling* yourself not to worry about results. Although you're focusing on a different precept than in Stage One, the method for allowing worry to fade is the same as it was for making it possible for anger to fade: *Just practice*. Recite the precepts. Do your energy practice/meditation. Give yourself Reiki every day without fail. Focus on your practice instead of on your worry.

If a worry does begin to arise, repeat the precept to yourself silently like a mantra, over and over, distracting your mind with it until the anxiety fades. Using the precept this way will help you in the moment and allow you to release each instance of worry. Devoting yourself fully to your practice helps worrying lessen more and more over time. Trust the practice, and give it time to work.

֍ Reiki for a pet three times per week (10 minutes)

Continue to give your pet or pets Reiki several times a week.

Here's how:

Give your pet Reiki when he or she is already resting comfortably.

Sit down next to your cat, or put him on your lap, and lay your hands on any spot you wish. If you know he has a painful place on his body, go ahead and put your hands there if you want. Otherwise, any spot that feels right to you is fine. Focus your attention on allowing energy to flow into the animal, and once you feel you have established that connection, forget about trying to do anything else.

Leave your hands on that one spot for ten minutes, or fewer, if your cat decides he's had enough and gets up and walks away. Picking just one spot to rest your hands gives you good practice at giving Reiki without trying to bring about a result. Just as when you're giving Reiki to people, this is a great opportunity to give all your attention to establishing and maintaining the energy connection with your pet.

�֍ **Weekly distant Reiki for someone else, preferably as a trade with a partner** (20 minutes)

In your work at this stage, you'll focus on different spots than you did in Stage One, and you'll also incorporate the new energy practice/meditation as a regular part of your distant Reiki session.

Doing the distant session:

- Do Gassho and mentally establish a connection with your partner, either imagining his or her body in front of you, or using a surrogate, such as a stuffed animal.

- Place your hands at the crown. As you start the session, also begin doing this variation on the Stage Two energy practice: inhale into your hara; then exhale and imagine the energy flowing out of your hara, up into your arms, down through your hands, and out to your partner. Remember to do the session without trying to effect any healing or outcome at all.

- After ten minutes, move your hands to the heart and give Reiki for ten more minutes.

- End the session by doing Gassho and then receiving Reiki from your partner, if you're working with one. Remember to do Gassho once more once both halves of the session are complete, and state your gratitude for having the opportunity to do this practice.

✳ **Weekly hands-on Reiki for someone else, preferably as a trade with a partner** (20 minutes)

For Stage Two practice, you'll incorporate the Stage Two energy practice/meditation and focus on your partner's crown and heart:

- Do Gassho with your partner, recite Usui Sensei's precepts, and express your gratitude for the opportunity to do this practice with each other. Do 15 minutes of the Stage Two energy practice/meditation with your partner. Then whoever will be receiving first can lie down on the table or sit in the chair for the session.

- Do Gassho and mentally establish a connection with your partner.

- Start the session at your partner's crown, and initiate the Stage Two energy practice/meditation: inhale into your hara; then exhale and imagine the energy flowing out of your hara, up into your arms, down through your hands, and out to your partner. Remember to do the session without trying to effect any healing or outcome at all.

- After ten minutes, move your hands, one at a time, to your partner's heart. You can reach this position by standing at your partner's side and laying your hands in a line (or one atop the other) just below the collar bone. Or, if you're standing at your partner's head when you have your hands on his or her crown, you can remain standing there and lay your hands in a V-shape, with the heels of your hands roughly on the shoulders and your fingers approaching each other to form a V. Give Reiki for ten more minutes.

- End the session with three head-to-toe sweeps above the body, and do Gassho toward your partner.

- Switch positions with your partner, so that you are the recipient.

When you've completed both sessions, end by doing Gassho toward each other and expressing your thanks for the opportunity to work with each other.

✠ Monthly instruction, attunements and discussion with a teacher (Optional)

If you are working with a teacher regularly as part of your practice, do take the time with him or her to review how you're doing. I meet with my students about once a month to check in, and hear about what benefits they're noticing, which parts of the practice are going smoothly, and which seem more challenging. Touching base with your teacher is a great way to review your work in the practice and to ask for feedback or suggestions about moving forward.

When to move on to Stage Three

Although it helps to discuss your work on this path with a teacher before moving to the next stage, you can certainly make this decision on your own. Reviewing what benefits you're receiving from your practice, as you did before beginning Stage Two Practice, will help you decide whether it's time to move ahead. Take a look at this list and see whether you are experiencing any of these positive effects:

- You find that your ability to focus during the energy practice/ meditation and the Reiki sessions has increased.

- The energy practice meditation flows easily.

- You are more aware of the energy flowing through your body.

- You are less distracted while giving or receiving Reiki.

- You look forward to giving yourself Reiki and notice that it helps you.

- You feel you are going more deeply into the session when you receive Reiki.

- People who receive Reiki from you tell you that it feels deeper, or that it feels like you're working on a different level, or they are experiencing more or deeper releases during and after sessions.

- You've noticed that your reflection on the precepts has helped you cope with difficult moments in your life.

- You are feeling more patient with yourself, others, and the practice.

- You are feeling happier.

- You feel little resistance to keeping to your routine.

- You've settled into a consistent practice and schedule.

- You find that it's easier to concentrate on what you're doing, both during practice and in other areas of your life.

- You feel more committed to the practice.

- You've found that using your practice has helped you when you're upset.

- You feel you're working hard on your practice and would like added challenge.

- You're enjoying the practice!

I'll bet that more than a few of these ring true for you. If that's the case, and you've been practicing at Stage Two for about a month or so, then it's appropriate for you to move to Stage Three.

Chapter Eight

Stage Three Practice: "Just for Today, Express Gratitude"

In this stage you'll be learning a new energy practice/meditation, a variation on which you'll then incorporate into all the Reiki sessions you give to others, including pets. You'll continue to use two hand positions when giving Reiki, but they will be slightly different than in previous stages. The differences in the practice elements are small, but they will make it possible for you to take your Reiki even deeper than you've done so far. I invite you to read on and acquaint yourself with what's new:

Stage Three Practice:

- Daily Gassho, followed by repeating Usui Sensei's Reiki precepts.

- Daily energy practice/meditation.*

- Daily self-Reiki.*

- Reflection on the third Reiki precept: "Just for today, express gratitude."*

- Reiki for a pet three times per week.

- Weekly distant Reiki with a partner, if you have one, or for someone else of your choosing.*

- Weekly hands-on Reiki with a partner, if you have one, or for someone else of your choosing.*

- Optional: monthly communication with a teacher, to discuss the practice and to receive an attunement.

Stage Three Practice, Step by Step

Begin each day with:

✠ Gassho, expressing gratitude, and repeating Usui Sensei's precepts

Put your hands in the Gassho position (with your hands in front of your chest, palms together,) close your eyes, and give thanks that you have the opportunity to do this practice that will benefit both you and others.

Next, while keeping your hands in Gassho, recite aloud the following phrases written by Usui Sensei. View this recitation as a way to sincerely offer your gratitude for having the opportunity, time and motivation to be doing this practice that has so much potential for benefitting you and those around you, to remind yourself of the purpose of this practice, and to set your intention to have ongoing awareness of the precepts Usui Sensei taught. Give your full attention to the words as you slowly repeat them:

> *The secret of inviting happiness through many blessings*
> *The spiritual medicine for all illness*
>
> *Just for today:*
> *Do not be angry*
> *Do not worry*
> *Express gratitude*
> *Devote yourself diligently to your work*
> *Be kind to people*
>
> *Do Gassho every morning and evening*
> *Repeat the precepts and keep them in your mind and heart*
> *To improve your body and mind*

Once you've done this recitation, do Gassho again and proceed to…

✠ Daily energy practice/meditation (15 minutes)

Do this energy practice/meditation each day after you recite the Reiki precepts. This stage's practice is a variation on what you already know.

The Stage Three energy practice/meditation:

First: Begin by doing the Stage Two energy practice/meditation for a minute or two: draw energy down into your hara as you inhale and sending it out through every cell of your body as you exhale.

Next: As you inhale, call to mind someone you love deeply, and pull this love-infused energy down through your heart into your hara. Just think of this person and allow your love to rise as you inhale and fill your hara. There's no need to force it or to think specific thoughts about the person. Simply call him or her to mind and allow loving feelings to arise as you breathe in.

Next: As you exhale, send energy out from your hara in all directions, and imagine that you are sending your love out to this person atop this energy that is flowing outward.

Summary: Think of someone you love as you inhale through your heart and into your hara, and send love to him or her along with the energy you send out as you exhale. Continue on in this way for about ten minutes.

Move from this energy practice right into…

Daily self-Reiki session (20 minutes)

Start the session by tuning in to what your body is telling you and let what you pick up guide your hand placements. The less often you move your hands, the better, so that you can go deeply into the session.

If you don't feel drawn to any particular spots when you tune in, try placing your hands at your heart, solar plexus or hara. Rest your hands on one of those spots for ten minutes. Then move to another spot and give yourself Reiki there for ten more minutes.

I also encourage you to integrate the Stage Three energy practice/meditation you've just learned into your self-Reiki sessions: once you have decided where to put your hands, begin doing the energy practice/meditation and continue with it for the entire twenty minutes.

As well, as you move to this new stage of practice, take a fresh look at your self-Reiki practice. Are you able to stay focused as you give yourself Reiki, and are you enjoying it, or is this part of your practice feeling stale, like a chore? If it's the latter, then adding in the energy practice/meditation should help. Also consider how many hand positions you're using. The less you move your hands around while giving yourself Reiki, the easier it will be for you to feel a deeper connection to the energy, so try using only two or three hand positions during each self-Reiki session.

✴ **Reflection on the third Reiki precept**: Just for today, express gratitude.

Usui Sensei's third precept has often been translated as "Just for today, be humble," but the original Japanese wording contains a set phrase that means "express gratitude." Certainly, gratitude is connected to humility. If we express gratitude for whatever we encounter in our lives, then humility also comes into play: being humble can mean admitting that maybe we do not know everything or understand everything in life well enough to be able to judge which circumstances might help or hinder us. Acknowledging this opens the door to feeling grateful for all that comes our way in life. So, let's begin our reflection on this precept by considering what we feel grateful for in our lives. I'll share some of my own thoughts on this with you.

Every day I express my gratitude for being able to practice: for having the resources and opportunity to learn from gifted teachers, the time to pursue my practice, and the chance to write this book. When I do Gassho, it is a gesture of my gratitude for the teachings, those who have taught me, those with whom I'm able to share Reiki in any way, and to Usui Sensei for offering us the Reiki teachings in the first place.

I am also grateful for my practice, because my ability to stay calm and to feel love and compassion for others is a fruit of the time and effort I pour into practicing.

When you experience similar moments of gratitude as you travel on this path of practice, that's a great time to do Gassho and consciously give thanks for the practice that is making a positive difference in your life, and to Usui Sensei for the original teachings.

Feeling grateful about other areas of our life can be more of a challenge. We might find that we devote a lot of energy to thinking about what we want, but don't have, whether it's a new car, a bigger house, a higher-paying or more enjoyable job, or more time with those we love, or a spiritual practice that will rid us of unhappiness. Or about what we *don't* want, but do have to put up with: higher taxes, annoying co-workers, chores to do on the weekend, being apart from those we love.

No matter whether we're focusing on what we do want or don't want, though, what lies at the root of our musings is dissatisfaction with the way our life is. When we're in this frame of mind, we're too busy worrying about why happiness hasn't come into our lives to concentrate on opening the door and inviting it in. One way we can break that cycle is to shift our focus and express our gratitude for all that is right.

So, take a sheet of paper, or use the blank pages in the back of this book, and make a list of what you feel grateful for in your life: concrete items, people in your life, circumstances, experiences you've had, or what you've learned. My list would definitely include losing my teaching job to budget cuts. I wasn't grateful for that on the day that happened, but I am now, since that's what enabled me to find my way to Reiki. You, too, might feel thankful for some of the most difficult experiences of your life.

As you add each new item to the list, give yourself time to think about it and enjoy whatever happiness might arise in connection with it. You can also note down *why* you're grateful for the people or events or experiences you're noting down.

Once the list is as long as you think it needs to be, take note of how you're feeling. I imagine that after making this list, you're feeling a least a little bit happy. Imagine how your happiness might increase if your gratitude grew. So, how do we make it possible to experience more gratitude? *Just practicing* will definitely help you feel more and more grateful for everything in your life. Thoughts of happiness and thankfulness will start bubbling up more and more, while dissatisfaction with your life will begin to lessen.

Also make use of the practice elements to help this process along: when you notice you're feeling dissatisfied something in your life, or find yourself complaining about the way things are, using the third precept as a mantra can help you refocus and express gratitude for whatever is going well. Giving yourself Reiki can also allow the dissatisfaction to fade away; so can expressing thanks for having this wonderful tool at your fingertips.

Finally, here's a meditation that will help gratitude arise and grow:

Expressing gratitude

Here's how:

- Look back at the list you just made. Now ask yourself, What could I do to express gratitude for this circumstance or person or occurrence? The point here is not to make an actual plan of action, but to brainstorm all possible ways to express your thanks, whether it's within the realm of possibility or not. For example, if I think about how I might express my gratitude to Usui Sensei for his teachings, I might decide to offer him a boundless field of wildflowers to represent the blossoming I've experienced by practicing Reiki. Or if I'm grateful to my friend for always lending an ear when I'm upset, I might want to bake her a fabulously delicious and beautifully decorated cake and drop it off at her house as a surprise. Or a mountain of cupcakes, or a pyramid of potted flowers that stretches up into the sky. You get the idea! So...

- Find a quiet space and set aside ten to fifteen minutes to devote to this meditation, whether after self-Reiki or the energy practice/meditation, or at some other time. Go down your list, item by item and imagine ways to express your gratitude. Take your time. Close your eyes, if it helps you focus. Use your imagination. Above all, have fun with it! Remember, the sky's the limit. You don't even need to write your ideas down. Just look at the list, and go from there.

- End your meditation by doing Gassho and expressing your gratitude for your practice.

Once you do this meditation a couple of times, you'll probably reach the end of your list. When that happens, you can either sit down and make a whole new list with new items, or you can vary the meditation: first call to mind someone or something for which you're grateful, and then imagine how you could express your gratitude. Go through this process several times in the course of one session.

I love this meditation, first of all because it's so fun: you get to think up amazing ways to express your thanks. In addition, simply going through this process infuses your mind with gratitude, and then you carry that feeling with you wherever you go afterwards. That's not all, though. Remember how I said back in Chapter Four that the Buddhists consider committing to observe precepts a very powerful action? It's the same with this meditation. Working in this way is like spending fifteen minutes affirming your devotion to allowing more and more gratitude to arise in your heart and mind.

Do this meditation whenever you want. Either save it for times when you're feeling a little dissatisfied, or make it part of your routine as you work your way through Stage Three. But do incorporate it into your regular routine because it really does jumpstart your gratitude and allow it to grow even more quickly.

And remember, the best way to help gratitude blossom in your heart is to … *just practice!*

※ Reiki for a pet three times per week (10 minutes)

For Stage Three Practice, you'll pick one part of your pet's body to work on for ten minutes, while incorporating a variation on your new energy practice/meditation.

To begin the session, choose one spot to concentrate on and mentally establish a connection with your pet. Once you've done so, begin using the energy practice/meditation: as you inhale, think of your pet with love, and allow that love to flow down through your heart and into your hara. As you exhale, pull this love-infused energy up and *send it out through your hands to your pet*. Continue for ten minutes, or as long as your pet wants to receive Reiki.

※ Weekly distant Reiki for someone else, preferably as a trade with a partner (20 minutes)

Do the distant Reiki sessions using a stuffed animal as a surrogate, or imagine your partner's body in front of you, whichever feels most comfortable to you.

What's new in this stage is that you'll be using a variation on the Stage Three energy practice/meditation as you send Reiki to your partner.

Doing the distant session:

- Do Gassho and mentally establish a connection with your partner, either imagining his or her body in front of you, or using a surrogate, such as a stuffed animal.

- Place your hands at the crown. As you start the session, also begin doing this variation on the Stage Three energy practice/meditation: Call to mind someone you love deeply (it can be someone other than the recipient!), and inhale, pulling the love down through your heart and into your hara. As you exhale, pull this love-infused energy up and *send it out through your hands to your partner*. Take your time and allow the energy to flow without forcing it. Also remember to do the session without trying to effect any healing or outcome at all.

- After ten minutes, move your hands to the heart and give Reiki for ten more minutes.

- End the session by doing Gassho and then receiving Reiki from your partner, if you're working with one. Remember to do Gassho once more when you've completed both halves of the session, and state your gratitude for having the opportunity to do this practice.

Weekly hands-on Reiki for someone else, preferably as a trade with a partner (20 minutes)

For Stage Three practice, you will begin as you've been doing all along, and then add in the variation on the energy practice/meditation:

- Do Gassho with your partner, recite Usui Sensei's precepts, and express your gratitude for the opportunity to do this practice with each other. Do 15 minutes of the Stage Two energy practice/meditation with your partner. Then whoever will be receiving first can lie down on the table or sit in the chair for the session.

- Do Gassho and mentally establish a connection with your partner.

- Start the session at your partner's crown and begin the same variation on the Stage Three energy practice/meditation that you're now using during your distant sessions with your partner: Call to mind someone you love deeply, and inhale, pulling the love down through your heart and into your hara. Then exhale, sending the love-infused energy *out through your hands to your partner*. Remember to take your time and to allow the energy to flow without forcing it. Just breathe at a natural, comfortable pace, and visualize the energy flowing gently in and out.

- After ten minutes, move your hands, one at a time, to your partner's heart and give Reiki for ten more minutes.

- End the session with three head-to-toe sweeps above the body, and do Gassho toward your partner.

- Switch positions with your partner, so that you are the recipient.

- When you've completed both sessions, end by doing Gassho toward each other and expressing your thanks for the opportunity to work with each other.

✴ Monthly instruction, attunements and discussion with a teacher (Optional)

Are you in contact with a teacher as you're working through this practice? If you are, be sure to check in with him or her to talk about how your practice is going, discuss any questions you have about the practice and to receive an attunement.

If you have not been working with a teacher, this would be a good time to try to arrange such a meeting. It can help you feel more confident that you are on the right track with your practice, and receiving regular attunements will give your practice a boost, too! You can look back at Chapter Three ("Preparing for Your Journey") for suggestions about how to find a teacher to work with.

After you've settled in to Stage Three practice, at some point you'll wonder when it would be appropriate to move to Stage Four. When you begin considering this, the first step is to ask yourself whether you're continuing to benefit from your practice. Do you feel these statements reflect your practice experience?

- You find that your ability to focus during the energy practice/ meditation and the Reiki sessions has increased.

- The energy practice meditation comes flows easily.

- You are more aware of the energy flowing through your body.

- You are less distracted while giving or receiving Reiki.

- You look forward to giving yourself Reiki and notice that it helps you.

- You feel you are going more deeply into the session when you receive Reiki.

- People who receive Reiki from you tell you that it feels deeper, or that it feels like you're working on a different level, or they are experiencing more or deeper releases during and after sessions.

- You've noticed that your reflection on the precepts has helped you cope with difficult moments in your life.

- You are feeling more patient with yourself, others, and the practice.

- You are feeling happier.

- You feel little resistance to keeping to your routine.

- You've settled into a consistent practice and schedule.

- You find that it's easier to concentrate on what you're doing, both during practice and in other areas of your life.

- You feel more committed to the practice.

- You've found that using your practice has helped you when you're upset.

- You feel you're working hard on your practice and would like added challenge.

- You're enjoying the practice!

If you are noticing more and more benefit from practicing, that's a good indication that you're ready to begin Stage Four Practice. It shows that you've gone deeply into what you have already been doing, and that's an excellent sign! But there's one more question to ask yourself as you're deciding whether to move on to Stage Four: how comfortable are you with the limited hand positions you've been using so far in the practice?

During the first three practice stages, you haven't been choosing where to put your hands, except during self-Reiki. Limiting the number of hand positions makes it easier for you to settle into giving Reiki in a way that becomes meditative and also allows you stay in that state, instead of repeatedly shifting out of it as you move your hands. Using two pre-determined positions also frees you from making a decision about where to place your hands. This also helps you sustain the meditative state and feel less distracted by any intuitive messages you may be receiving.

This ability to stay focused on giving Reiki to your partner without giving in to distractions is a key aspect of your practice and all of the elements help you grow more skillful at this. Ideally, by the time you've been doing Stage Three practice for a while, you will find that you are able to give distant or hands-on Reiki without being overwhelmed by impulses to move here or there during a session, and without the strong desire to go to a certain spot so you can fix or heal your partner. It's not that the intuitive information or impulses are not there — because you may still receive that kind of information. Rather, when you do realize something about your partner's physical or emotional state, your concentration doesn't get broken by your desire to respond to what you're noticing in your partner.

If you are pretty comfortable at staying in the two places indicated for each stage of practice, and if you find you're not distracted by intuitive information, then by all means, go on to Stage Four. (In Stage Four, you'll have the freedom to choose your hand positions, although you'll still be limited to two!) If not, then it's better to stay at Stage Three until you are feeling totally comfortable with this way of giving Reiki has faded.

CHAPTER NINE

Stage Four Practice:
"Just for Today, Devote Yourself Diligently To Your Work"

What's new in this stage, aside from the focus on Usui Sensei's fourth precept, is that you will finally choose two places to lay your hands during distant and hands-on Reiki!

Stage Four Practice:

- Daily Gassho, followed by repeating Usui Sensei's Reiki precepts.

- Daily energy practice/meditation.

- Daily self-Reiki.

- Reflection on the fourth Reiki Precept: "Just for today, devote yourself diligently to your work."*

- Reiki for a pet three times per week.

- Weekly distant Reiki with a partner, if you have one, or for someone else of your choosing.*

- Weekly hands-on Reiki with a partner, if you have one, or for someone else of your choosing.*

- Optional: monthly communication with a teacher, to discuss the practice and to receive an attunement.

Stage Four Practice, Step by Step

Begin each day with:

✠ Gassho, expressing gratitude, and repeating Usui Sensei's precepts

Put your hands in the Gassho position (with your hands in front of your chest, palms together,) close your eyes, and give thanks that you have the opportunity to do this practice that will benefit both you and others.

Next, while keeping your hands in Gassho, recite aloud the following phrases written by Usui Sensei. View this recitation as a way to sincerely offer your gratitude for having the opportunity, time and motivation to be doing this practice that has so much potential for benefitting you and those around you, to remind yourself of the purpose of this practice, and to set your intention to have ongoing awareness of the precepts Usui Sensei taught. Give your full attention to the words as you slowly repeat them:

> *The secret of inviting happiness through many blessings*
> *The spiritual medicine for all illness*
>
> *Just for today:*
> *Do not be angry*
> *Do not worry*
> *Express gratitude*
> *Devote yourself diligently to your work*
> *Be kind to people*
>
> *Do Gassho every morning and evening*
> *Repeat the precepts and keep them in your mind and heart*
> *To improve your body and mind*

Once you've done this recitation, do Gassho again and proceed to…

❇ Daily energy practice/meditation (15 minutes)

Continue with the Stage Three energy practice/meditation:

First: Begin by doing the Stage Two energy practice/meditation for a minute or two: draw energy down into your hara as you inhale and sending it out through every cell of your body as you exhale.

Next: As you inhale, call to mind someone you love deeply, and pull this love-infused energy down through your heart into your hara. Just think of this person and allow your love to rise as you inhale and fill your hara. There's no need to force it or to think specific thoughts about the person. Simply call him or her to mind and allow loving feelings to arise as you breathe in.

Next: As you exhale, send energy out from your hara in all directions, and imagine that you are sending your love out to this person atop this energy that is flowing outward.

Summary: Think of someone you love as you inhale through your heart and into your hara, and send love to him or her along with the energy you send out as you exhale. Continue on in this way for about ten minutes.

Move from this energy practice right into...

Daily self-Reiki session (20 minutes)

Start the session by tuning in to what your body is telling you and let what you pick up guide your hand placements. The less often you move your hands, the better, so that you can go deeply into the session.

If you don't feel drawn to any particular spots when you tune in, try placing your hands at your heart, solar plexus or hara. Rest your hands on one of those spots for ten minutes. Then move to another spot and give yourself Reiki there for ten more minutes.

I also encourage you to integrate the Stage Three energy practice/meditation you've just learned into your self-Reiki sessions. Once you have decided where to put your hands, begin doing the energy practice/meditation: Think of someone you love as you inhale through your heart and into your hara, and send love to him or her along with the energy you send out as you exhale. Continue on in this way for the entire session.

Reflection on the Fourth Reiki Precept: Just for today, devote yourself diligently to your work.

Usui Sensei's fourth precept has often been translated as "Do your work honestly" and "Be honest in your work." However, a Japanese speaker explained that this is not precisely what the precept's Japanese transliteration, *gyoo hagemu*, conveys. Although the noun *gyoo* can have many meanings, when combined with the verb *hagemu*, it suggests "calling, vocation, business, trade or profession." The verb itself expresses the idea of "applying or devoting oneself assiduously." So, although Usui Sensei would undoubtedly have encouraged his students to work honestly, the essence of the precept lies in the idea of focused, devoted attention to a task. Usui Sensei was encouraging us to devote ourselves not to just any work, but to our calling, in other words, *to our practice.*

If we view Usui Sensei's precepts as the commitments we make to travel on the transformative path that a Reiki practice offers us, then reciting the fourth precept reminds us that when we choose to devote ourselves to practicing Reiki, we are doing more than taking up a hobby. We're expressing our faith in Reiki's ability to help us transform our lives and enable us to help others, too.

When we feel drawn to throw ourselves wholeheartedly into this endeavor, we embrace a goal that is focused not on achieving concrete, material results, or status or power or admiration, or on satisfying our own everyday desires, but on being able to benefit others by transforming our own heart and mind. When this motivation is present, our practice becomes a calling. I believe Usui Sensei was urging us to work in precisely this way.

By beginning this precept with the words "devote yourself diligently," Usui Sensei was telling us that if we want our practice to truly transform our lives and invite in happiness, then we have to keep at it. Both this precept and Usui Sensei's instructions to repeat the precepts and keep them in our mind and heart remind us that allowing benefit to arise from the practice takes consistent, devoted, assiduous work.

So now, as you embark on Stage Four Practice and reflect on this precept, devote some time to taking stock of your practice and reviewing your routine.

What motivates you to practice?

At the beginning of Stage One Practice, I asked you to consider why you were beginning this practice. If you still have your answers to those questions, read over them now. Then take a sheet of paper (or use the back of the book) and make some notes about what is motivating you *now* to continue devoting yourself to this practice.

Did you answer this question differently than when you were first starting out? My students have. At the beginning of Stage One, they spoke in general terms: they wanted to grow spiritually, or feel more open, or develop a regular practice. When I asked them at the beginning of Stage Four what kept them motivated, they replied: "Now I'm getting more from the Reiki. And when I'm doing Reiki, I'm more focused and not distracted." "I'm more aware of when anger is growing, and I can release it." "It's so profound that I can't find the words." "I'm more aware of what I'm trying to overcome." "The energy is always there." "Because of the benefits, I'm happy to continue."

In other words, as practitioners go deeper into the practice, they're inspired to keep going not by a hope that something in their lives will change, but by the actual transformation they're already noticing, and by the desire to invite even more happiness into their lives. That's natural: seeing positive change arise as a result of your efforts gives your practice a giant boost, because the benefits show you that you're on the right track. This is one of the biggest pluses of practicing: devote yourself fully, and the joy you experience will motivate you to keep up your practice.

Is anything holding you back?

You probably wouldn't be reading this chapter if you weren't seeing benefits from your practice. Even so, outside circumstances and our own personality and tendencies can sometimes make it difficult for us to devote ourselves to our practice as fully as we might like to do. Take a moment now and consider whether you would like to be putting more time into practice than you currently are. If the answer is yes, then this is a good time to try to get a handle on what might be making it difficult for you to do that.

There are a number of reasons you aren't able to practice as diligently as you'd like to be doing. Here are some possibilities to consider:

- Are there so many demands on your time and energy that you find it difficult to fit in all the practice elements? If so, take a look at your commitments and consider which ones you can let go of to free up some time for practice. Cutting back on other activities can be difficult, but simplifying your life in this way will definitely benefit your practice.

- Even if you can't free yourself up from any of your other commitments, think about which of them you can rearrange to make your practice times more consistent.

- Is your practice partner consistent and reliable? A partner who tends to cancel or who frequently asks to reschedule your meetings will throw practice off for both of you. If this is the case for you, talk with your partner about how important it is to you to keep to your scheduled practice times.

Even if you feel everything with your practice is going perfectly now, reviewing your routine now is a wonderful way of working with the fourth precept: it reaffirms your commitment to your practice and allows you to adjust any elements that have gotten a bit off track.

❈

Another way to go more deeply into your understanding of the fourth precept is to consider what "devote yourself diligently to your work" might mean for you personally, aside from sticking to your practice routine. Take this opportunity to reflect more broadly on what being committed to your practice — or to any other activities in your life you might consider a calling — means to you. How does your commitment manifest itself, whether in your thoughts or actions? As always with these exercises, you can use a sheet of paper or the back of the book, or simply think about this question, either while you sit quietly, or during formal meditation.

As you continue to work through Stage Four Practice, continue to consider how you can bring this precept to bear, in both your Reiki practice and your life in general.

❈ Reiki for a pet three times per week (10 minutes)

To begin the session, choose one spot to concentrate on and mentally establish a connection with your pet. Once you've done so, begin using the energy practice/meditation: as you inhale, think of your pet with love, and allow that love to flow down through your heart and into your hara. As you exhale, pull this love-infused energy up and *send it out through your hands to your pet*. Continue for ten minutes, or as long as your pet wants to receive Reiki.

❈ Weekly distant Reiki for someone else, preferably as a trade with a partner (20 minutes)

What's new in the Stage Four distant Reiki session is that you'll actually be deciding on the two spots to concentrate on during the session! Finally, a little freedom!

Doing the distant session:

- Do Gassho as usual, and mentally establish a connection with the recipient.

- With your hands in Gassho, establish a connection with your partner and silently express your openness to becoming aware of what areas of your partner's body would like Reiki. This is similar to what you've been doing all along during self-Reiki, but now you'll bring this approach to work with your partner. Wait for a few moments until you gain a sense of where it might be good to put your hands. Sometimes this information will come to you as a thought or impression. Sometimes you may feel as sensation in your own body or an emotion that seems to be coming from the recipient. Once you receive some indication of this type, just decide on two spots you'll focus on. You'll begin with one and stay there for ten minutes, and then switch to the other. If you don't feel drawn to any particular area, that's not a problem. You can simply stick with the crown, heart or hara.

The main thing is to pick your spots and don't change your mind during the session! As always, your task is simply to connect with your partner and give Reiki, not to focus on bringing about any result.

- As you begin the session, also begin using this variation on the Stage Three energy practice: Call to mind someone you love deeply, and inhale, pulling the love down through your heart and into your hara. As you exhale, pull this love-infused energy up and send it out through your hands to your partner. Continue on in this way for about ten minutes

- While continuing to do this energy practice/meditation, give your partner Reiki, spending ten minutes at each of the two spots you picked at the beginning of the session.

- End the session by doing Gassho and then receiving Reiki from your partner, if you're working with one. Remember to do Gassho once more once both halves of the session are complete, and state your gratitude for having the opportunity to do this practice.

⌘ Weekly hands-on Reiki for someone else, preferably as a trade with a partner (20 minutes)

- Begin your time with your partner as you're used to doing, by doing Gassho, repeating the precepts and spending 15 minutes on the energy practice/meditation.

- Once your partner is in position to receive Reiki from you, put your hands in Gassho, and establish a connection with him or her.

- As you have your hands in Gassho, silently express your openness to becoming aware of what areas of your partner's body would like Reiki. Based on what you become aware of, choose two hand positions for the session.

- Start the session at the first position of your choice.

- Once you feel the energy begin to move through you, begin the variation of the Stage Three energy practice/meditation: Call to mind someone you love deeply, and inhale, pulling the love down through your heart and into your hara. Then exhale, sending the love-infused energy *out through your hands to your partner.*

- Work this way for ten minutes, and then move your hands, one at a time, to the second spot you've chosen, while continuing with the energy practice/meditation. Give Reiki at this spot for ten more minutes.

- End the session with three head-to-toe sweeps above the body, and do Gassho toward your partner.

- Switch positions with your partner, so that you are the recipient.

- When you've completed both sessions, end by doing Gassho

toward each other and expressing your thanks for the opportunity to work with each other.

Monthly instruction, attunements and discussion with a teacher (Optional)

Continue to check in with your teacher for guidance about your practice and to receive an attunement.

How long should you stay at Stage Four? If, after practicing at this stage for a month or two, you feel very comfortable choosing spots, and don't find that you become distracted by information you pick up from your partner, then it's fine to move on to Stage Five.

CHAPTER TEN

Stage Five Practice: "Just for Today, Be Kind to People"

In this stage, you'll learn a new energy practice/meditation, which you'll incorporate into your hands-on and distant Reiki. You'll also be lengthening your sessions, which will help you go deeper into your practice.

Stage Five Practice:

- Daily Gassho, followed by repeating Usui Sensei's Reiki precepts.

- Daily energy practice/meditation.*

- Daily self-Reiki.*

- Reflection on the fifth Reiki Precept: "Just for today, be kind to people."*

- Reiki for a pet three times per week.*

- Weekly distant Reiki with a partner, if you have one, or for someone else of your choosing.*

- Weekly hands-on Reiki with a partner, if you have one, or for someone else of your choosing.*

- Optional: monthly communication with a teacher, to discuss the practice and to receive an attunement.

Stage Five Practice, Step by Step

Begin each day with:

�֎ **Gassho, expressing gratitude, and repeating Usui Sensei's precepts**

Put your hands in the Gassho position (with your hands in front of your chest, palms together,) close your eyes, and give thanks that you have the opportunity to do this practice that will benefit both you and others.

Next, while keeping your hands in Gassho, recite aloud the following phrases written by Usui Sensei. View this recitation as a way to sincerely offer your gratitude for having the opportunity, time and motivation to be doing this practice that has so much potential for benefitting you and those around you, to remind yourself of the purpose of this practice, and to set your intention to have ongoing awareness of the precepts Usui Sensei taught. Give your full attention to the words as you slowly repeat them:

The secret of inviting happiness through many blessings
The spiritual medicine for all illness

Just for today:
Do not be angry
Do not worry
Express gratitude
Devote yourself diligently to your work
Be kind to people

Do Gassho every morning and evening
Repeat the precepts and keep them in your mind and heart
To improve your body and mind

✣ Daily energy practice/meditation (20 minutes)

The energy practice/meditation for this stage has two parts.

First: As you inhale, think of *someone you love*, and allow the love you feel to fill your heart. As you exhale, allow that love to flow outward from your heart, without withholding it or trying to keep any of it in.

Next: On the next inhale, think of someone *who loves you*. Allow yourself to breathe that person's love into your heart and fill it. As you exhale, allow that love to flow out of you, without clinging to it.

Continue this cycle, first feeling your love for others, and then allowing yourself to accept others' love.

Do this meditation for 20 minutes (instead of the 15 you've been used to).

Move from this energy practice right into…

�֎ **Daily self-Reiki session** (20 minutes)

Start the session by tuning in to what your body is telling you and let what you pick up guide your hand placements. The less often you move your hands, the better, so that you can go deeply into the session.

If you don't feel drawn to any particular spots when you tune in, try placing your hands at your heart, solar plexus or hara. As you give yourself Reiki, incorporate the new energy practice/meditation:

First: As you inhale, think of *someone you love*, and allow the love you feel to fill your heart. As you exhale, allow that love to flow outward from your heart, without withholding it or trying to keep any of it in.

Next: On the next inhale, think of someone *who loves you*. Allow yourself to breathe that person's love into your heart and fill it. As you exhale, allow that love to flow out of you, without clinging to it.

Continue using the energy practice/meditation throughout your session.

✖ **Reflection on the Fifth Reiki Precept**: Just for today, be kind to people.

Here we are at Usui Sensei's fifth precept. This precept's Japanese wording is not a lofty, spiritual expression conveyed in lofty, spiritual language, but rather, a common, everyday phrase: "be kind to people." Yet, as familiar and ordinary as this phrase may be, here it is, in the final position on Usui Sensei's list. Did he place it last because being kind to people is so easy, and so commonsense a notion that we barely need to be reminded to do it? I don't think so. This may, in fact, be the most difficult precept to put into action. If that's the case, why is it at the end of the list?

We can see the precepts as a description of what we can achieve as we practice: first our anger and worry begin to fade, then it becomes easier for us to make headway with the last three precepts. As we grow more skillful at not being swept away by anger, our mind is not so disturbed, and we worry less. This means it's easier for us to be grateful for our life circumstances, easier to concentrate on our calling, and easier to be kind to others.

Perhaps you've begun to experience this as a benefit from your own practice. If you find you're feeling kinder toward people, that's because your sincere and diligent practice has made it possible for anger and worry to fade and for positive emotions to gradually take their place.

You can describe this process another way: as your positive emotions grow, you invite more and more happiness into your life, and you naturally begin sharing your happiness with everyone around you. That's what lies at the heart of Usui Sensei's final precept: being kind to others means fully and joyfully sharing all the love and happiness that you yourself are feeling with everyone around you.

This might seem a natural way to behave, but it's not necessarily easy to pass all your happiness along in the form of kindness to others. In the course of our daily lives, even if we are feeling loving or filled with happiness, we might also have lingering resentments or doubts or anxieties which cause us to hold back from being as kind and loving as we might otherwise be. Or perhaps we're afraid of losing others' love or affection, so we try to hoard those happy feelings in some way, storing them up so we can draw on them if our supply is somehow cut short. Feeling this kind of anger or worry can make it difficult for us to share our own happiness and send a full stream of love and kindness to those around us.

But it's this very act of sharing our own happiness, fully and sincerely, which completes the cycle of inviting more happiness into our lives — and others'. If, when great happiness arises in us, we don't pass it on, it's like slamming the door to happiness instead of inviting it in. Our practice opens a doorway, an opening that's meant to allow happiness and love to flow through in *both* directions. That's why, when we notice that happiness has begun to flow our way, our task is to make sure we are doing all we can to send just as much of it as possible back out into the world. This is another way of understanding what Usui Sensei meant by "be kind to people": invite them to accept happiness from you.

How, then, do you nurture your ability to share your happiness with others, without withholding it? You'll grow better at being able to share your happiness with others by using the same method that's helped you invite happiness into your own life: *Just practice*. Trust that if you keep devoting yourself to your practice, your ability to pass along your own happiness will grow. Your sincere practice has brought you this joy, and it will help you pass it along, too. So, keep practicing.

This stage's new energy practice/meditation will help you, too, since it gives you regular practice at sending love out without holding any of it back. Use this meditation when you find yourself in a situation where you're not feeling inclined to share your happiness. You don't even need to close your eyes: just think of someone you love and imagine sending love to them. Then imagine love coming back from them.

Your main task, though, as always, is to keep practicing. Let your practice do the work.

� Reiki for a pet three times per week (10 minutes)

To begin the session, choose one spot to concentrate on and mentally establish a connection with your pet. Once you've done so, begin using the new energy practice/meditation: the first time you inhale, think of someone you love, and allow the love you feel to fill your heart. As you exhale, allow that love to flow outward from your heart, without withholding it or trying to keep any of it in. The next time you inhale, think of someone who loves you. Allow yourself to breathe that person's love into your heart and fill it. As you exhale, allow that love to flow out of you, without clinging to it. If you wish, you can make one of your animals the focus of the meditation during the sessions.

Use this energy practice/meditation throughout your session for your pet.

� Weekly distant Reiki for someone else, preferably as a trade with a partner (30 minutes)

In this stage, you and your partner will be incorporating the new energy practice/meditation into thirty-minute sessions.

The second change is that now you and your partner will give each other distant Reiki for 30 minutes, instead of the 20 you've been used to. You'll continue to choose your hand positions, but since the sessions will be longer now, you can either use two hand positions, for 15 minutes each, or pick three positions at the beginning of the session and spend 10 minutes at each.

Doing the distant session:

- Do Gassho as usual, and mentally establish a connection with the recipient.

- With your hands in Gassho, establish a connection with your partner and silently express your openness to becoming aware of what areas of your partner's body would like Reiki. Wait for a few moments until you gain a sense of where it might be good to put your hands. Once you receive some indication of this type, just decide on either two or three spots to focus on. (If you pick two spots, you'll stay at each for fifteen minutes; if you pick three, you'll stay at each for ten minutes.)

- As you begin the session at the first position you've chosen, also begin using this variation on the Stage Five energy practice: the first time you inhale, think of someone you love, then as you exhale, send that love out through your hands to your partner. The second time, inhale while thinking of someone who loves you and allow that love to flow into you, and as you exhale, send that love out through your hands to your partner. It's perfectly okay if the person you call to mind, the person you love, is not your practice partner! What's important is to allow feelings of love to arise in your heart and to send those loving feelings out during your Reiki session, and then, to allow yourself to be replenished by allowing love to flow in from someone in the second half of the practice.

- While continuing to do this energy practice/meditation, give your partner Reiki, spending ten minutes at each of three spots, or fifteen minutes at each of two spots.

- End the session by doing Gassho and then receiving Reiki from your partner, if you're working with one. Remember to do Gassho once more once both halves of the session are complete, and state your gratitude for having the opportunity to do this practice.

Weekly hands-on Reiki for someone else, preferably as a trade with a partner (30 minutes)

Your hands-on sessions, just like your distant sessions, will now be 30 minutes long, and you can choose either 2 or 3 hand positions. You'll also be incorporating this stage's new energy practice/meditation.

Doing the session:

- Begin your time with your partner by doing Gassho, repeating the precepts and spending fifteen minutes on the energy practice/meditation.

- Once your partner is in position to receive Reiki from you, put your hands in Gassho, and establish a connection with him or her.

- As you have your hands in Gassho, silently express your openness to becoming aware of what areas of your partner's body would like Reiki. Based on what you become aware of, choose either 2 or 3 hand positions for the session.

- Start the session at the first position of your choice.

- Once you feel the energy begin to move through you, begin this variation on the new energy practice meditation: the first time you inhale, think of someone you love; then, as you exhale, send that love out to your partner through your hands. The second time you inhale, think of someone who loves you and allow that love to flow into you. As you exhale, send that love out through your hands to your partner.

- Work this way for fifteen minutes (or ten, if you've chosen 3 hand positions,) and then move your hands, one at a time, to the next spot you've chosen, while continuing with the energy practice/meditation. If you've decided to focus on three hand positions, move your hands again after ten minutes.

- End the session with three head-to-toe sweeps above the body, and do Gassho toward your partner.

- Trade sessions in the usual way, ending by doing Gassho toward each other and expressing your thanks for the opportunity to work with each other.

Monthly instruction, attunements and discussion with a teacher (Optional)

If you are working with a teacher, continue to check in with him or her to discuss how your practice is going and to receive an attunement. If you have not been working with a teacher, it's not too late to start! Maybe it's been a while since you looked for someone to help you move through the practice, so it couldn't hurt to give it another try.

The first person to approach is the teacher who trained you in Reiki. He or she might be interested in serving as a resource for you as you practice. If that's not possible or doesn't feel like the right fit for you, don't hesitate to ask your Reiki-trained acquaintances whether they think their teacher might enjoy helping you with the practice. It's definitely worth asking around, and even consulting with a number of teachers.

If you do find a teacher who is interested, it's important for him or her not only to support you in your practice, but to also be supportive of the practice framework itself. So, the most important question to ask a prospective teacher is how comfortable he or she is with the practice framework. After all, if you've chosen to devote yourself to this practice, you want a teacher who also feels positive about it, so that you can receive as much benefit as possible.

❧

Although we've come to the end of Usui Sensei's list of precepts, there is one more practice stage ahead. You could continue working at the current stage of practice indefinitely, since there is no limit to how much you can develop your ability to share your happiness with others. Whenever you feel that you've settled in with Stage Five Practice — you find it easy to use the energy practice/meditation both on its own and during your Reiki sessions, and have adjusted to the longer sessions — feel free to start on the next stage, which will help you go deeper into your practice.

CHAPTER ELEVEN

Stage Six Practice: "Just for Today"

If you're reading this chapter, then you've probably been engaging in the Heart of Reiki practice for quite a while. So, I'm very happy to see you here, and to introduce you to new variations on the elements you're already familiar with:

Stage Six Practice:

- Daily Gassho, followed by repeating Usui Sensei's Reiki precepts.

- Daily energy practice/meditation.

- Daily self-Reiki.

- Reflection on the Reiki Precepts: "Just for today."*

- Reiki for a pet three times per week.

- Weekly distant Reiki with a partner, if you have one, or for someone else of your choosing.*

- Weekly hands-on Reiki with a partner, if you have one, or for someone else of your choosing.*

- Optional: monthly communication with a teacher, to discuss the practice and to receive an attunement.

Stage Six Practice, Step by Step

Begin each day with:

�֎ Gassho, expressing gratitude, and repeating Usui Sensei's precepts

Put your hands in the Gassho position (with your hands in front of your chest, palms together,) close your eyes, and give thanks that you have the opportunity to do this practice that will benefit both you and others.

Next, while keeping your hands in Gassho, recite aloud the following phrases written by Usui Sensei. View this recitation as a way to sincerely offer your gratitude for having the opportunity, time and motivation to be doing this practice that has so much potential for benefiting you and those around you, to remind yourself of the purpose of this practice, and to set your intention to have ongoing awareness of the precepts Usui Sensei taught. Give your full attention to the words as you slowly repeat them:

> *The secret of inviting happiness through many blessings*
> *The spiritual medicine for all illness*
>
> *Just for today:*
> *Do not be angry*
> *Do not worry*
> *Express gratitude*
> *Devote yourself diligently to your work*
> *Be kind to people*
>
> *Do Gassho every morning and evening*
> *Repeat the precepts and keep them in your mind and heart*
> *To improve your body and mind*

❖ Daily energy practice/meditation (20 minutes)

First: As you inhale, think of *someone you love*, and allow the love you feel to fill your heart. As you exhale, allow that love to flow outward from your heart, without withholding it or trying to keep any of it in.

Next: On the next inhale, think of someone *who loves you*. Allow yourself to breathe that person's love into your heart and fill it. As you exhale, allow that love to flow out of you, without clinging to it.

Continue this cycle, first feeling your love for others, and then allowing yourself to accept others' love.

Do this meditation for 20 minutes.

Move from this energy practice right into…

❖ Daily self-Reiki session (20 minutes)

Start the session by tuning in to what your body is telling you and let what you pick up guide your hand placements.

As you give yourself Reiki, incorporate the Stage Five energy practice/meditation:

First: As you inhale, think of *someone you love*, and allow the love you feel to fill your heart. As you exhale, allow that love to flow outward from your heart, without withholding it or trying to keep any of it in.

Next: On the next inhale, think of someone *who loves you*. Allow yourself to breathe that person's love into your heart and fill it. As you exhale, allow that love to flow out of you, without clinging to it.

Continue using the energy practice/meditation throughout your session.

❊ Reflection on the Reiki Precepts: Just for today

As you've made your way through all the practice stages, you've focused on each of the precepts in turn, taking your understanding of them deeper and reflecting on what each of them means to you within the context of your life. In this chapter, let's talk about how we can interpret "Just for today." I say "we", because I want to stress that although each of us is engaging in our own, individual practice, we are also all practicing together, motivated and guided by the same principles. In this way we serve as a continual support for each other in this shared endeavor, both every day and *just for today*.

We might assume that because Usui Sensei introduced his precepts with this phrase, he was urging us to take direct, daily action to figure out a way not to get angry; to consciously keep worry from our minds; or to consider exactly how we can go about increasing our gratitude, or our motivation, or our compassion. Rather, Usui Sensei encouraged his students to repeat the precepts very day and keep them in their mind and heart. As well, he taught his students to practice Reiki so that they could feel a deep connection with the recipient. He gave them a practice framework that would, if they engaged wholeheartedly in that practice, help this feeling of connection grow, and allow happiness to arise. So, as I see it, "Just for today" tells us not *what to do*, but rather *how* to practice. ·

Part of that "how" involves being diligent: "Just for today" reminds us that our practice is an ongoing process, that our task on any given day — and on *every* day — is to devote ourselves sincerely to this endeavor. Our daily practice lays the groundwork for the transformations we will undergo, so these words remind us of our commitment to the day-to-day work that will facilitate the changes within us.

"Just for today" also encourages us to exercise patience. We engage in this work because we hope our suffering will fade and our happiness will grow, preferably *right now*! Sometimes it's very difficult to be patient. So, "Just for today" tells us, "The way to see progress is to patiently give the practice your full attention right now, here, today." Just for today, because our efforts in this moment build the strong foundation of our future happiness. So, we give our full attention to practicing and not to thoughts about what changes we hope to see in our lives.

As we continue with our practice, Usui Sensei's words let us know that we might experience one or more of these benefits "just (for) today," or to varying degrees. Some days we will feel angry and worried, some days we will feel grateful and motivated, and some days we will feel like we are riding a roller coaster moving back and forth between those two extremes. Usui Sensei understood that we are not perfect, so "Just for today" tells us not to expect to be bundles of sunshine twenty-four hours a day.

In fact, it's quite natural to feel ups and downs as we continue with our practice. We see our minds change little by little, but that doesn't mean that we are always at the same level of calm or gratitude or motivation. Our emotions flow like a river, that is sometimes high and sometimes low. There are dry spells, as well as periods when the river is like a raging torrent. The emotions in our mind are no different: we might find that calm and turbulence alternate.

What matters is how we respond when these varying emotions arise. When we feel great happiness and recognize it as a benefit of our practice, we might think, "Yes!! Now I've got it!! I'm home free!" When strong anger arises, we might conclude that we've utterly failed at our practice and might as well give up. The trick when this happens is to notice what we're experiencing, but not to conclude that our practice is finished — in either the positive or negative sense! — as a result. Recognize that although we're exhilarated today, we might not be tomorrow. Although we're angry today, we might feel exhilarated tomorrow, because it can work that way, too! In other words, whatever we're feeling is "just for today," and tomorrow's experience may or may not be the same.

Remembering this can be a great relief, because it can help us not be distracted by the thought that we're doing something wrong. We can say to ourselves, "Wow! Today is tough!" We can note it and give ourselves a little more Reiki, and *just practice*. When we're really, really happy, we can allow ourselves to soak up that joy, let it sink in a little deeper and then share it with those around us.

At this point, maybe you're thinking, "But if I'm really happy, can't I *do* something to keep myself happy, and if I'm angry, can't I *do* something to make it not come back again?" You sure can. *Just practice*. Throughout the six stages of this practice, you've been learning to do that: to give or receive Reiki without expecting or looking for a certain outcome. It's the same with the practice as a whole. The way to allow the benefits of the practice to arise — the benefits the precepts express — is to express gratitude for the chance to engage in this practice, to devote yourself sincerely and diligently to it, and to recognize, with kindness, that there is more anger and worry that can fade, as well as more gratitude, kindness and happiness ahead. In other words, *Just practice. Just for today. Just for every day.* That'll do it.

�֍ Reiki for a pet three times per week (10 minutes)

To begin the session, choose one spot to concentrate on and mentally establish a connection with your pet. Once you've done so, begin using the new energy practice/meditation: the first time you inhale, think of *someone you love*, and allow the love you feel to fill your heart. As you exhale, allow that love to flow outward from your heart, without withholding it or trying to keep any of it in. The next time you inhale, think of someone *who loves you*. Allow yourself to breathe that person's love into your heart and fill it. As you exhale, allow that love to flow out of you, without clinging to it. If you wish, you can make one of your animals the focus of the meditation during the sessions.

Use this energy practice/meditation throughout your session for your pet.

✖ Weekly distant Reiki for someone else, preferably as a trade with a partner (30 minutes)

Although you'll be giving distant Reiki just as you did in Stage Five — 30 minute sessions, with 2 or 3 hand positions, incorporating the

Stage Five energy practice/meditation (which I'll review with you be-low) — now, you and your partner will both send Reiki simultaneously. In other words, you will be *simultaneously* sending and receiving Reiki.

My students didn't know what to expect when they first began giv-ing distant Reiki this way, but once they tried it, they reported that they felt this new method actually helped them go deeper into each session. They felt they received even more benefit from distant Reiki than they had before. So, try it, and see what happens!

Doing the distant session:

- Follow these instructions and give your partner distant Reiki. At the same time, remember that he or she will simultane-ously be giving distant Reiki to you. Enjoy!

- Do Gassho as usual, and mentally establish a connection with the recipient.

- With your hands in Gassho, establish a connection with your partner and silently express your openness to becoming aware of what areas of your partner's body would like Reiki. Wait for a few moments until you gain a sense of where it might be good to put your hands. Once you receive some indication of this type, just decide on either two or three spots to focus on. (If you pick two spots, you'll stay at each for fifteen minutes; if you pick three, you'll stay at each for ten minutes.)

- As you begin the session at the first position you've chosen, also begin using this variation on the Stage Five energy prac-tice: the first time you inhale, think of someone you love, then as you exhale, send that love out through your hands to your partner. The second time, inhale while thinking of someone who loves you and allow that love to flow into you, and as you exhale, send that love out through your hands to your partner. It's perfectly okay if the person you call to mind, the person you love, is not your practice partner! What's important is to allow feelings of love to arise in your heart and to send those loving feelings out during your Reiki session, and then, to al-low yourself to be replenished by allowing love to flow in from someone in the second half of the practice.

- While continuing to do this energy practice/meditation, give your partner Reiki, spending ten minutes at each of three spots, or fifteen minutes at each of two spots.

- End the session by doing Gassho, and state your gratitude for having the opportunity to do this practice.

✷ Weekly hands-on Reiki for someone else, preferably as a trade with a partner (30 minutes)

You and your partner will continue to give each other 30 minute sessions, focusing on either 2 or 3 hand positions. The partner *giving* Reiki will do so exactly as you did in Stage Five. The difference at this stage is that the partner who is on the *receiving* end of the session will also do the Stage Five energy practice/meditation while receiving Reiki. So, as you are lying on the table (or sitting in a chair) when it's your turn to receive, do the energy practice/meditation the entire time. (If you work with a volunteer who is not a Heart of Reiki practitioner, he or she can receive in his or her usual way, and you can do the energy practice/meditation when it's your turn to receive.)

As you're receiving Reiki in this way, you may become so relaxed that you just drop off to sleep or feel too relaxed to continue the practice. That's okay! You don't need to resist that, if it happens. Just do the practice as long as you can while receiving.

Doing the session:

- Begin your time with your partner by doing Gassho, repeating the precepts and spending fifteen minutes on the energy practice/meditation.

- Once your partner is in position to receive Reiki from you, put your hands in Gassho, and establish a connection with him or her.

- With your hands in Gassho, silently express your openness to becoming aware of what areas of your partner's body would like Reiki. Based on what you become aware of, choose either 2 or 3 hand positions for the session.

- Start the session at the first position of your choice.

- Once you feel the energy begin to move through you, begin this variation on the Stage Five energy practice meditation: the first time you inhale, think of someone you love, then as you exhale, send that love out to your partner through your hands. The second time you inhale, think of someone who loves you and allow that love to flow into you. As you exhale, send that love out through your hands to your partner.

- Work this way for fifteen minutes (or ten, if you've chosen 3 hand positions,) and then move your hands, one at a time, to the next spot you've chosen, while continuing with the energy practice/meditation. If you've decided to focus on three hand positions, move your hands again after ten minutes.

- End the session with three head-to-toe sweeps above the body, and do Gassho toward your partner.

- Trade sessions in the usual way, ending by doing Gassho toward each other and expressing your thanks for the opportunity to work with each other.

✳ Monthly instruction, attunements and discussion with a teacher (Optional)

Continue to check in with your teacher for guidance about your practice and to receive an attunement.

What comes next?

Up until now, there has always been a next stage to move onto once you've decided you're ready to take that step. What about now? What should you do after you've settled into Stage Six and have been working with those elements for a month, or two, or three? *Keep going!*

During these six stages, you've learned a practice framework that has remained pretty constant in its elements, except for the evolving energy practice/meditation and each stage's focus on a different precept. I imagine that you've grown more and more comfortable with practicing Reiki in this new way that may have seemed unfamiliar at the start. I hope that at this point you can reflect on your life and see that you are receiving some of the benefits that Usui Sensei mentions in his precepts, and that you feel you have been inviting more and more happiness into your life. If you do, then your practice is definitely facilitating the transformation that lies at the heart of Reiki.

You may also feel that more happiness is waiting to flow into your heart and your life, that more transformation is possible. Certainly, there is no limit to the happiness that can arise out of your practice, and so, there is no end point to the Heart of Reiki practice. I ended the book with Stage Six because once you've come this far, you can keep practicing with the elements you've already learned, and continue to experience ongoing and deeper transformation. Once you've settled into the Stage Six practice, the best course of action is continue on with that framework and allow what you already know to evolve.

This is exactly what happened in my own work with Reiki. Once I'd completed my Reiki Master Teacher training, it was by throwing myself into Reiki as my life's work , that my Reiki practice deepened and evolved alongside my Buddhist practice. I didn't set out to transform my Reiki practice into the framework I teach you here. But that's what developed as I devoted myself consistently and seriously to this work.

Similarly, the key for you is to move ahead with the awareness that this is a practice you can use for your entire life. Approach it with diligence and patience, just as you are doing now, and allow the practice to evolve, without looking for specific results. By all means, keep working with your partner and your teacher; the whole practice framework as a unit is what has brought you the benefits you've already noticed. So, keep up with all of it.

As you move ahead, you will probably feel more motivated to practice at some times and less at others. Don't worry about that. At times when you're feeling less enthusiastic, here are some suggestions for ways to boost your practice:

- Give yourself more Reiki.

- Go back and look at the energy practices/meditations for the various stages, and focus on one of them for a week or two.

- Review the precepts and do the same reflections you did at various stages. Spend some time on the precept that seems most challenging to you at the moment. If you're feeling stuck or unmotivated, going through the exercise on gratitude in Stage Three can really give you a boost!

- Look back at the section in Chapter Five ("Gauging Your Progress") that helps you determine whether you're making progress with your practice. This can help you feel confident that you're still on the right track.

Really, the main thing as you move forward is, as always, to *Just practice!* and see what happens. You've gotten very good at doing that, so continue to trust yourself and your practice: let the practice do the work of inviting happiness into your life.

There is something else you can do to help your practice deepen, though, that doesn't involve learning any new techniques or practice elements: you can begin integrating some of the practice elements into any Reiki sessions you're doing outside of your practice time. Maybe you've already begun doing that, either consciously or without realizing it. In the next chapter I'll give you specific suggestions about how to go about that.

CHAPTER TWELVE

The Heart of Reiki In Your Professional Practice

There's no specific point when it's right to begin integrating what you're practicing into your informal or professional Reiki sessions. In fact, you may already have begun doing so without realizing it. But here's a general guideline: if you feel well-settled into your own practice, and if you notice that you personally are benefiting from it, then it's perfectly appropriate to begin incorporating what you have learned into your Reiki work with others. Doing so will allow them to experience even greater benefits when receiving Reiki from you, and your own practice will also deepen. This chapter explains how combining your personal and professional practices can be good for everyone; how to prepare recipients so that they'll receive the most benefit from these sessions; and how to integrate the practice elements into your sessions.

Everyone benefits

You began this practice in the hope that you would experience personal or spiritual transformations that would invite happiness into your life. Recall that Usui Sensei made this possible for his students by giving them the opportunity to share Reiki with each other over and over again. This enabled them to feel steadily more strongly connected to each other. As they experienced this connection, they grew more loving and compassionate and thus, happier. Sharing their joy with others, they began to feel even greater happiness themselves.

I imagine that as you've engaged in this practice, you've found yourself becoming happier and calmer. It's the consistent flow of energy you and your partner establish by giving and receiving Reiki with gratitude, focused attention and compassion — the heart of Usui Sensei's method — that makes this growing happiness possible.

The practice routine you've developed ensures a regular cycle of giving and receiving Reiki, and this cycle is key to allowing happiness to arise. Since you both give and receive Reiki regularly, you can relax into the giving without worrying that you won't be receiving Reiki, or without being angry — even ever so slightly — that you don't get Reiki as often as you'd like. You may not have considered this consciously before, but think about it: before you began this practice, maybe you received Reiki only intermittently. So, each time a session ended, you may have felt a twinge of sadness that it was over, particularly if you didn't know when you'd have another session. Rather than being able to climb lightly and willingly off the Reiki table, you may have resisted getting up, because you wanted to lie there and soak up the wonderful feeling, hoping it would carry you over until the next time some Reiki came your way.

This is a pretty subtle psychological moment, that moment at the end of a session when you either resist and think, "No! I don't want it to end!" or smile and sit up, ready to move on, whether it's to giving Reiki to your friend or heading out the door. Receiving Reiki regularly and frequently means that it gradually becomes easier for you to relax and enjoy Reiki, instead of feeling a little sad or angry that the session is over. So, your practice routine actually helps you observe the first two precepts: Just for today, do not be angry. Just for today, do not worry.

This benefit of your ongoing practice is not only enjoyable; it's absolutely key to the process of developing deep love and compassion for those around you: although any dissatisfaction at a session's end may be subtle, it can still distract you and make it difficult for you to be fully open and giving when it's your turn to offer Reiki to your friend. When this happens, your mind is permeated by wanting, instead of giving. By engaging in the Heart of Reiki practice, though, you begin to relax. You gradually become less reluctant to get up after your own session, and happier to give your partner Reiki. In other words, your state of mind becomes steadily more oriented toward giving. This helps your love grow, which in turn invites more and more happiness into your life.

You've also been helping this process along by doing the Stage Five energy practice/meditation: you first imagine sending love out from your heart, without withholding any bit of it, and then allow love to flow into you, but without clinging to it. This alternating flow of love, out and in, in and out, mirrors the feelings you experience when giving and receiving Reiki with your partner. Believe it or not, practicing this meditation will make it easier to climb off the table without regret and give Reiki without feeling grudging about it.

Being able to receive Reiki without feeling sorry to have it end, and give Reiki with a sincere, open heart, is one of the biggest benefits you can experience from your ongoing practice. When your own practice is sustaining, and happiness is flowing into your life, the impulse to give becomes ever more deeply ingrained in you; you grow more giving in your life as a whole. It's at this point, when you feel a growing orientation toward giving, that your professional recipients will begin to benefit more from your practice than they've done before. That's the best time to consciously begin integrating the practice elements into those Reiki sessions, because now, giving Reiki to others becomes a way of sincerely sharing your own happiness with them.

Approaching your work for other recipients this way gives you the opportunity to practice sending out love and comfort even if you are not, in the moment, expecting to receive that in return. You are actively sharing the happiness and gratitude and compassion that have arisen in you by offering others Reiki with loving attention just because you have the opportunity to do so. Each Reiki session you give, then, reinforces your habit of giving of yourself freely and lovingly and invites more happiness into your life. Sharing the fruits of your experience in this way both deepens your practice and brings profound benefits to others.

Now let's look at specific ways you can help your recipients enjoy the transformative benefits of all the marvelous work you've been doing in your practice!

�֎

Although you'll now begin using certain practice elements in your non-practice sessions, there are some differences between giving Reiki in these two settings. In your practice, you use Reiki and the energy practice/meditations not to bring about healing, but to maintain the energy flow that's necessary for facilitating personal or spiritual transformation. But when clients or friends come to you for Reiki, they're usually looking for relief from an ailment or stress or anxiety. When you're giving Reiki in these cases, it's easy to find yourself focusing on an outcome, no matter how long you've been doing your own practice. But if you move out of the frame of mind in which you've been giving Reiki as part of your practice, this reawakened focus on a result will limit both your Reiki practice and your recipients' benefit. So, let's see how you can find a middle ground between the extremes of treating a session as if it were just another practice meeting with your partner, or falling back into the habit of trying to figure out what's wrong and make it better. You'll do this by adjusting both how you present the session to recipients and how you yourself approach giving Reiki to others.

A new way of talking with recipients

Shifting the way you talk about Reiki can help your recipients begin to be open to experiencing transformation in their lives. The key is to gently encourage them to simply receive the Reiki without expectations and "see what happens". Here are some ways to help you get that message across:

- Be careful with the word "healing." If you describe giving Reiki as providing healing, then both you and recipients can slip into assuming that you, the practitioner are giving healing to them, the passive receiver. Speaking of a Reiki session as a step in a transformative process is a useful way to talk about what goes on during sessions. Tell recipients that Reiki gives them energy that their mind and body can use to help them experience personal transformation. That way everyone can see the sessions as the collaborative effort they truly are.

- Start by asking recipients what's brought them to you for Reiki. Their answers will tell you whether or not they have a specific outcome in mind. Sometimes clients will say that they've heard of Reiki and want to see what it can do for them. If that's the case, affirm that this kind of openness is wonderful. Say that you've found this "try it and see what happens" approach very beneficial.

When, on the other hand, recipients express hope that their pain or anxiety will disappear during a session, I start by telling them they may very well experience relief during the session. Then I say that if they can go into the session with that "try it and see what happens" attitude, then they might end up receiving relief from a worry or condition they weren't even thinking about. I encourage them to relax and invite the energy in without hoping for a given outcome. Some people are more receptive to this idea than others, so with those who seem resistant, be gentle, but do your best to help them enter the session without the expectation that they will walk out cured of whatever is ailing them.

- You've grown accustomed to offering Reiki without an intent to cure or heal, and you'll do so in these non-practice session, but still do ask recipients whether they have any pain or discomfort. You're asking not because you intend to try to fix anything, but so that you can be aware of what is going on with the recipient. Having you ask will help them feel cared about and taken care of, and indeed, tell them that during the session, you will probably place your hands where their discomfort is. That will feel soothing to them.

- After the session, there's no need to discuss what you may or may not have noticed with the recipient. That's mainly because as you're giving Reiki, your focus will be on connecting and being present, just as it is when you work with your practice partner, not on gathering information about the person's condition. When your recipients do ask what you noticed during a session, you might respond in one of these ways: "I wasn't trying to pick up anything. I find I'm able to go more deeply into giving you the energy when I just focus on the connection and on being with you." Or "I was drawn to put my hands on your shoulders, and it just felt right to stay there for a long time." In other words, let recipients know that you're focusing on just being there with them, instead of trying to figure out or fix something. They will appreciate your devotion to what you're doing.

- Definitely do encourage recipients to come for Reiki regularly. Talking with people about how often to have Reiki can be awkward, because you don't want them to feel pressured. But one big plus of your own practice experience is that you can talk to clients about the benefits of ongoing Reiki sessions. Here's one way I sometimes explain this: "Receiving Reiki regularly keeps your energy flowing and makes deep releases and transformations possible, so the more frequently you come for a session, the more you will benefit." You can also mention the transformations you are seeing from your own practice and explain that regular Reiki facilitates this kind of change. By talking with recipients about Reiki in this way, you help them learn to approach their sessions as something like a regular practice, too. When they see how your work with Reiki has helped you, they're likely to be more receptive to making Reiki a regular part of *their* lives.

Integrating the practice elements into your sessions

Now let's talk about how to adjust the way you give Reiki sessions so that recipients can begin to experience deeper benefits.

What's most important in this regard is to do what you always do when giving Reiki: establish a strong energetic connection with the recipient and offer Reiki with loving intent, without being distracted by the desire to act on thoughts or intuitive information that pass through your mind. Here are some specific suggestions for using your practice elements to enhance Reiki sessions for your clients or other recipients:

- Before beginning a session, spend 5-10 minutes doing the energy practice/meditation of your choice. I recommend the Stage Five meditation, because it reinforces the idea of alternating giving and receiving. This gets your energy flowing more strongly and also helps you settle into the meditative state, so that you'll be less distracted by outer stimuli or by thoughts and impulses that arise during the session.

- Once your recipient has settled in for the session, do Gassho, and then, with your hands still in Gassho, close your eyes. Establish a connection to him or her and be open to becoming aware of spots on his or her body that would like attention:

Stand at the recipient's head or side, do Gassho, and ask to become aware of which parts of the body would like attention. Do this with your hands on his or her head, or do a scan of the body if you wish. (Starting at the crown, with your hands 4-5 inches about the head, move your hands slowly along the length of the body, from head to toe, and notice whether any spots attract your attention. Make sure to do this without touching the body.) As you move your hands above the body, you may feel drawn to concentrate on certain spots. Once you have identified two or three such spots, begin your session.

I suggest choosing your hand positions before you begin the session so that you don't have to try to decide that as you're going along. If you do this, you'll be able to maintain a stronger connection with the recipient, since you won't be repeatedly thinking about where you should put your hands next.

- For the same reason, limit the number of hand positions you use during the session. Every time you move your hands, you're pulling your attention away from maintaining the energy connection with your recipient. It's your focus and sustained connection that allows the recipient to go deeply into a session.

- Do place your hands on spots that you think will bring comfort to the recipient! This is one big difference between giving Reiki to your practice partner and to other recipients. I taught you not to move your hands during practice sessions so that you would develop the ability to maintain your connection to your partner without being distracted by other stimuli, whether external or in the form of information you were picking up from your partner. But now that you've gotten better at staying focused, it's appropriate to *notice* where you feel your hands might be most welcome and to put them there, because you definitely do want your recipient to feel comforted! But still limit the amount you move: strike a balance between staying put and responding to what you are noticing about your recipient.

Here's one way to do this: pick a spot that seems right to you, then allow yourself to settle in fully, as if you're forgetting that you might ever move your hands again. Don't move them again until you really feel drawn to do so. If that means that you spend the entire session working at only a couple of spots, that's fine. The key is to maintain the connection and not move your hands every two minutes in response to a thought or impression or image that enters your head. This is one of the biggest challenges in giving Reiki to others, but you've been honing this skill in your own practice, so definitely bring it to bear now, with your recipients.

- No matter where you do put your hands during the session, remember to give Reiki without expectations, just as you've been doing for yourself and your practice partner. This is the other big challenge you'll face when integrating The Heart of Reiki into other sessions. The first time you use this approach during a non-practice session you might well feel awkward, or worry that if you're not focused on actively bringing healing to your recipients, then you're letting them down, that you're somehow *not* facilitating healing. This is not at all the case. In fact, you are opening the door for them to benefit even more than before, because you are intent only on connecting with them with love, being present, and offering them energy. So, think of the sessions as offering recipients energy and love that they can use in their own transformative process; then you will probably not worry so much. (If necessary, remind yourself of Usui Sensei's second precept as you give Reiki!)

When I began giving Reiki to my clients this way, they noticed a difference, although I didn't tell them I was doing anything new. One of my regular clients told me that although receiving Reiki from me had always been a profound experience, now he felt it was much deeper and more profound than it had been before. I saw this as a wonderful affirmation of the value of my practice and of sharing it with recipients. So, trust the practice as you offer Reiki in this new way.

One final note: as you do begin integrating your Heart of Reiki practice into sessions for people other than your practice partner, continue to be diligent about your own practice. It's your devotion to your own practice that makes it possible for you to experience the benefits you are now able to help others receive, too.

I hope these guidelines will help you feel confident and joyful about sharing the fruits of your practice with those to whom you give Reiki. May you and your recipients receive the gift of ever-growing happiness. Gassho.

APPENDIX

Summary of Practice Elements for Each Stage

Here you'll find a brief description of the practice at each of the six stages. It's meant to serve as shorthand to help you remember your practice elements, so that you don't have to look back to individual chapters, unless you want to review instructions in detail.

Stage One Practice

✠ **Gassho and expressing gratitude**: Do Gassho and recite precepts daily.

✠ **Daily energy practice/meditation**: Start with 10 minutes, then work up to 15 minutes.

As you inhale: Imagine energy flowing into your hara and collecting there.

As you exhale: Allow the energy to rest in your hara.

✠ **Daily self-Reiki session**: 20 minutes. Pick a spot; move when you feel drawn to do so. Use energy practice/meditation during the session if you feel distracted.

✠ **Reflection on the first Reiki precept**: Just for today, do not be angry

✠ **Reiki practice on animals three times per week**: 10 minutes or more

✠ **Weekly distant Reiki**: 10 minutes at *crown*, 10 minutes at *hara*. Use energy/practice/meditation if you feel distracted.

✠ **Weekly hands-on Reiki trade**: 20 minutes per person.

Gassho and recite precepts.

10-15 minutes of energy practice/meditation with partner before sessions

10 minutes at crown, 10 minutes at hara, while doing variation on energy practice/meditation: pull energy into hara as you inhale, then send out through your hands to your partner as you exhale.

Gassho at end.

❋

Stage Two Practice

❂ **Gassho and expressing gratitude**: Do Gassho and recite precepts daily.

❂ **Daily energy practice/meditation**: 15 minutes

As you inhale: Imagine energy flowing into your hara and collecting there.

As you exhale: Send energy out through your entire body.

❂ **Daily self-Reiki session**: (Same as in Stage One) 20 minutes. Pick a spot; move when you feel drawn to do so. Use energy practice/meditation as you practice if you feel distracted.

❂ **Reflection on the first Reiki precept**: Just for today, do not worry

❂ **Reiki practice on animals three times per week**: 10 minutes or more

❂ **Weekly distant Reiki**: 10 minutes at *crown*, 10 minutes at *heart*, while doing variation on Stage Two energy/practice/meditation: pull energy into hara as you exhale, send it out through your hands to partner as you exhale.

❂ **Weekly hands-on Reiki trade**: 20 minutes per person.

Gassho and recite precepts.

10-15 minutes of energy practice/meditation together before beginning sessions

10 minutes at *crown*, 10 minutes at *heart*, while doing variation on Stage Two energy practice/meditation: pull energy into hara as

you inhale, then send out through your hands to your partner as you exhale.

Gassho at end.

Stage Three Practice

🞅 **Gassho and expressing gratitude**: Do Gassho and recite precepts daily.

🞅 **Daily energy practice/meditation**: 15 minutes

As you inhale: Think of someone you love; allow energy to flow through heart to hara.

As you exhale: Send love-infused energy out through your entire body.

🞅 **Daily self-Reiki session**: 20 minutes, while doing Stage Three energy practice/meditation.

🞅 **Reflection on the third Reiki precept**: Just for today, express gratitude

🞅 **Reiki practice on animals three times per week**: 10 minutes or more, while doing Stage Three energy practice.

🞅 **Weekly distant Reiki**: 10 minutes at *crown*, 10 minutes at *heart*, while doing Stage Three energy practice.

🞅 **Weekly hands-on Reiki trade**: 20 minutes per person.

Gassho and recite precepts.

10-15 minutes of energy practice/meditation together before beginning sessions

10 minutes at *crown*, 10 minutes at *heart*, while doing Stage Three energy practice/meditation.

Gassho at end.

Stage Four Practice

✠ **Gassho and expressing gratitude**: Do Gassho and recite precepts daily.

✠ **Daily energy practice/meditation**: (Same as in Stage Three) 15 minutes.

As you inhale: Think of someone you love and allow energy to flow through heart to hara.

As you exhale: Send love-infused energy out through your entire body.

✠ **Daily self-Reiki session**: (Same as in Stage Three) 20 minutes, while doing Stage Three energy practice/meditation.

✠ **Reflection on the third Reiki precept**: Just for today, devote yourself diligently to your work.

✠ **Reiki practice on animals three times per week**: (Same as in Stage Three) 10 minutes or more, while doing Stage Three energy practice/meditation.

✠ **Weekly distant Reiki**: 10 minutes at *each* of two spots of your choosing, while doing Stage Three energy practice/meditation.

✠ **Weekly hands-on Reiki trade**: 20 minutes per person.

Gassho and recite precepts.

10-15 minutes of energy practice/meditation together before beginning sessions.

10 minutes at *each* of two spots of your choosing, while doing Stage Three energy practice/meditation.

Gassho at end.

Stage Five Practice

- **Gassho and expressing gratitude**: Do Gassho and recite precepts daily.

- **Daily energy practice/meditation**: 20 minutes.

First breath cycle: Inhaling, think of someone you love, and allow love for that person to fill your heart; exhaling, allow love to flow outward without withholding any of it.

Second breath cycle: Inhaling, think of someone who loves you and allow that love to fill your heart; exhaling, allow that love to flow out of you, without clinging to it.

- **Daily self-Reiki session**: 20 minutes, while doing Stage Five energy practice/meditation.

- **Reflection on the third Reiki precept**: Just for today, be kind to people.

- **Reiki practice on animals three times per week**: 10 minutes or more, while doing Stage Five energy practice/meditation.

- **Weekly distant Reiki**: 30 minutes total, with 15 minutes at *each* of two spots or 10 minutes at each of three spots of your choosing, while doing Stage Five energy practice/meditation.

- **Weekly hands-on Reiki trade**: 30 minutes per person.

  Gassho and recite precepts.

  15 minutes of energy practice/meditation together before beginning sessions.

  15 minutes at *each* of two spots or 10 minutes at each of three spots of your choosing, while doing Stage Five energy practice/meditation.

  Gassho at end.

Stage Six Practice

✠ **Gassho and expressing gratitude**: Do Gassho and recite precepts daily.

✠ **Daily energy practice/meditation**: (Same as in Stage Five) 20 minutes.

First breath cycle: Inhaling, think of someone you love, and allow love for that person to fill your heart; exhaling, allow love to flow outward without withholding any of it.

Second breath cycle: Inhaling, think of someone who loves you and allow that love to fill your heart; exhaling, allow that love to flow out of you, without clinging to it.

✠ **Daily self-Reiki session**: (Same as in Stage Five) 20 minutes, while doing Stage Five energy practice/meditation.

✠ **Reflection on the third Reiki precept**: Just for today.

✠ **Reiki practice on animals three times per week**: (Same as in Stage Five) 10 minutes or more, while doing Stage Five energy practice/meditation.

✠ **Weekly distant Reiki**: Give and receive Reiki *simultaneously*. 30 minutes total, with 15 minutes at *each* of two spots or 10 minutes at each of three spots of your choosing, while doing Stage Five energy practice/meditation.

✠ **Weekly hands-on Reiki trade**: 30 minutes per person. Same as Stage Five for the giver. Recipient does Stage Five energy practice/meditation while receiving.

Gassho and recite precepts.

15 minutes of energy practice/meditation together before beginning sessions.

15 minutes at *each* of two spots or 10 minutes at each of three

spots of your choosing, while doing Stage Five energy practice/meditation. Recipient does Stage Five energy practice/meditation while receiving.

Gassho at end.

ABOUT THE AUTHOR

Susan Downing grew up in Northern Illinois and went to college in Madison, Wisconsin, where she fell in love with Russian language and literature. This prompted her to earn her PhD in Slavic Languages and Literatures from the University of California at Berkeley. She taught Russian for more than 30 years and spent many cold, but heartwarming months studying and teaching in Russia and the former Soviet Union.

Susan stepped onto the path of her second career, as a Reiki practitioner and teacher, when she learned Reiki to enhance her volunteer work with hospice patients. At the same time, her Tibetan Buddhist practice was deepening, and in 2007, she took bodhisattva vows, thereby dedicating her life to helping others end their suffering. Susan quickly realized that working with Reiki complemented her Buddhist practice, and embraced Reiki as the focus of her bodhisattva work. While living a life of Buddhist and Reiki practice, she discovered a way to work with Reiki that enabled her to both deepen her own spiritual practice and connect more profoundly and joyfully with her students, clients and co-practitioners in Reiki. She drew on these discoveries to develop the Heart of Reiki practice she now shares with others.

In addition to Buddhism and Reiki, Susan enjoys cooking, hiking and reading. But most of all, she feels blessed to be able to spend time with her marvelous children, family and friends, who bring great richness and joy to her life.

Susan welcomes questions and comments from readers. You can contact her through her website:
www.MountainZendoAndHealingCenter.com